Teacher, Take Care

A Guide to Well-Being and Workplace Wellness for Educators

Edited by Jennifer E. Lawson

with Shannon Gander, Richelle North Star Scott, and Stanley Kipling

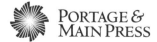

PORTAGE & MAIN PRESS

Text © 2022 Jennifer E. Lawson, Keith Macpherson, Laura Doney, Dana Fulwiler Volk, Shannon Gander, Monika Rosney, Richelle North Star Scott, Megan Hunter, Cher Brasok, Lisa Dumas Neufeld, Sandra Pacheco Melo, Jackie Gagné, Joyce Sunada, and Kelsey McDonald

Illustrations © 2022 Portage & Main Press

Portage & Main Press gratefully acknowledges the financial support of the Province of Manitoba through the Department of Sport, Culture, and Heritage and the Manitoba Book Publishing Tax Credit, and the Government of Canada through the Canada Book Fund (CBF) for our publishing activities.

Printed and bound in Canada by Friesens
Cover design by Jen Lum
Interior design by Relish New Brand Experience
Reviewer: Dr. Dorothy Young
Illustrations by Susan Kao

Library and Archives Canada Cataloguing in Publication
Title: Teacher, take care : a guide to well-being and workplace wellness for educators / edited by Jennifer E. Lawson with Shannon Gander, Richelle North Star Scott, and Stanley Kipling.
Names: Lawson, Jennifer, 1959- editor. | Gander, Shannon, editor. | Scott, Richelle North Star, editor. | Kipling, Stanley, editor.
Description: Includes bibliographical references.
Identifiers: Canadiana (print) 20220210837 | Canadiana (ebook) 20220211000 | ISBN 9781774920299 (softcover) | ISBN 9781774920305 (EPUB) | ISBN 9781774920312 (PDF)
Subjects: LCSH: Teachers—Mental health. | LCSH: Teachers—Health. | LCSH: Well-being. | LCSH: Work-life balance. | LCSH: Job stress. | LCSH: Stress management.
Classification: LCC LB2840 .T43 2022 | DDC 371.1001/9—dc23

25 24 23 22   1 2 3 4 5

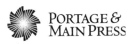

www.portageandmainpress.com
Winnipeg, Manitoba
Treaty 1 Territory and homeland
of the Métis Nation

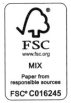

FSC
www.fsc.org
MIX
Paper from
responsible sources
FSC® C016245

ENVIRONMENTAL BENEFITS STATEMENT
Portage & Main Press saved the following resources by printing the pages of this book on chlorine free paper made with 30% post-consumer waste.

TREES	WATER	ENERGY	SOLID WASTE	GREENHOUSE GASES
34 FULLY GROWN	2,700 GALLONS	15 MILLION BTUs	110 POUNDS	14,800 POUNDS

Environmental impact estimates were made using the Environmental Paper Network Paper Calculator 4.0. For more information visit www.papercalculator.org

*This book is dedicated to teachers everywhere—
those who taught us, those who are friends and colleagues,
and those who have collectively changed the world.
May you always take care.*

Contents

Acknowledgements

For my part in this book, I will be eternally grateful to my first teachers, my amazing parents, Isabelle and Norm Lawson. They taught me, through their commitment to community and social justice, to always take care.—*Jennifer E. Lawson*

Heartfelt thanks to our courageous writers for your willingness to open your hearts and share your stories in support of teachers everywhere. And to the many educators I have worked with over the years who have taught me the true definition of resilience.—*Shannon Gander*

What a wonderful experience it has been for me to be part of this collaboration with such beautiful people. Thanks.—*Elder Stanley Kipling*

From my heart, I want to deeply acknowledge all my spiritual teachers (human and non-human alike), the ones in the past (my Ancestors), the present, and the future (the children). Whether you were aware of the impact you made or not, I have been blessed learning from you.—*Richelle North Star Scott*

Thank you, teachers, for holding our future in your hands. This work that you do is more important than you can ever know.—*Laura Doney*

I am forever grateful to be part of the teaching profession and want to thank my colleagues and fellow educators for their dedication and heart. You matter, your well-being matters, and you are appreciated. And thank you to all our family and friends who unconditionally uplift us along the journey.—*Dana Fulwiler Volk*

I would like to thank all my friends, family, and the many teachers who have inspired and encouraged me along the way. May this book arrive for you perfectly on time!—*Keith Macpherson*

I would like to honour and acknowledge my Creator, my family (especially my son, Luke), and all the mentors, helpers, healers, Knowledge Keepers, and Elders who have guided me on this journey. I am forever grateful.—*Lisa Dumas Neufeld*

I would like to acknowledge the land I was born on, Treaty 6 territory. Its nature is a gift that has shaped me and is why I began working in the field of health. A most heartfelt thank you to the brilliant humans who have been my guiding lights: Jenn Carson, the Health Advisors Huddle, the Joyful Collective, and my Mum. —*Megan Hunter*

How wonderful it's been to be part of this collaboration! The wellness of our educators is precious and important.—*Cher Brasok*

Much thanks to Guy, Kimmy, Lindsey, Melanie, Jane, Jennifer, M.J., and Marilyn for your constant support.—*Joyce Sunada*

I'd like to acknowledge my brilliant and passionately creative colleagues who continuously inspire and foster wellness through arts experiences.—*Jackie Gagné*

Thank you for the land and love grounding me; for my family, especially Chris, for supporting my wellness and writing; and for the students, families, and colleagues who have shared their wisdom.—*Monika Rosney*

With the encouragement of my family and Jennifer's support, this adventure has been a joy and honour. My gratitude for Genevieve, whose arrival in my life was a mysterious gift from the universe, is eternal. Without you, lady, I might still be in the basement with the band.—*Kelsey McDonald*

To my family, friends, staff, and colleagues, who remind me to take care of my mind, body, and spirit. I am grateful for you.—*Sandra Pacheco Melo*

Blessing

Elder Stanley Kipling

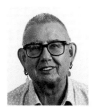

Elder Stanley Kipling, Dip FNCW, BSW, MSW, RSW, is a proud Peguis First Nation individual. Stan has extensive experience in areas related to Indigenous diversity, health-care issues in Indigenous populations, improving Indigenous cultural awareness, spiritual care, suicide prevention, addictions, anger management, family violence prevention, life skills, and personal development. Stan was raised on the trap line, hunting, commercial fishing, and living on the land. Stan is a Sundancer and Pipe Carrier, as well as a traditional harvester of animals and plants, and he has held Sweat Lodges.

I want to call on the Great Spirit, Gitchee Manitou, to bring blessings to this book and to the people who have contributed to the writings. It is with a warm heart and an open mind that I ask Creator to help each and every person who reads these writings for comfort and guidance in some way. Creator knows our hearts and struggles, and I ask for guidance for us all, in a good way, to the parts of the book that will speak to us.

Indigenous People are told that when we work with people who are struggling, we must speak from the heart. I believe that this book will speak to the hearts of many.

Introduction

Shannon Gander and Richelle North Star Scott

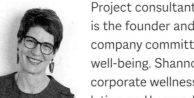

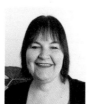

Project consultant **Shannon Gander**, BPE, CAC, CM, is the founder and director of Life Work Wellness, a company committed to individual and organizational well-being. Shannon has an academic background in corporate wellness, mental health, and conflict resolution, and has worked in the mental health community as a therapist and trainer since the early 1990s. For many years, she travelled Manitoba as part of the Balance team, bringing mental health program resources to educators. Shannon advocates for leaders to create systems for psychological health and safety for employees at all organizational levels. Her bliss is her family, nature, and a hot cup of coffee on a Saturday morning.

Knowledge Keeper and writer **Richelle North Star Scott** (Giiwedinong Anong) says Aniin! I am of Anishinaabe and Métis descent, and my Ancestors are from St Peter's Reserve. I am the mother of three beautiful daughters: Amanda, Tehya, and Riel. I am a KooKoo of a fabulous grandson named Darius, but I call him Noozhis (which means grandchild). I am the Coordinator of Indigenous Inclusion Education for the St James-Assiniboia School Division. I am a Mide woman, Pipe Carrier, Water Carrier, and Sundancer. I have completed my mystery* in land-based education. (*I don't use "master," as it is a gender-binary word.)

Welcome! You may have picked up this book because you want to know more about how to care for yourself. Or you may be wondering about someone else in your life. Perhaps you have concerns about educator burnout in your school. Regardless of why you chose this book, we are glad that you did.

Teacher, Take Care is an invitation to explore self-awareness and self-care for teachers, while also exploring workplace wellness on a larger scale. It invites us to consider how we can contribute to a culture that promotes and prioritizes the health and well-being of educators. When we engage in our self-care, we permit others to do the same. However, self-care alone will not prevent teacher burnout. We must look beyond the individual and focus on a systems-level approach to well-being at work.

Across the globe, organizations are exploring ways to embed psychological health and safety into their workplaces to protect employee mental health. There has been extensive research on the psychosocial factors that contribute to workplace well-being, including work-life balance, psychological support, and organizational culture. By taking actions to bolster these psychosocial factors in our schools, not only do we support the health of teachers but we also create healthier learning environments for students. Expanding workplace health and safety to include protection of mental wellness has been a long time coming. In chapter 13, "An Invitation for Leaders in Education," we look at the research and describe a systems-level approach to well-being for school leaders who want to take intentional actions to create healthy workplace environments. We encourage leaders at all levels to build systems that support our educators.

How to Use This Book

Teacher, Take Care is an interactive guide to help educators promote their personal well-being and workplace wellness. Within these pages, you will find opportunities to reflect and respond to questions. You may choose to simply think about the reflection questions, or you may record your journey. For example, you might keep a notebook-style journal or a sketchbook for visual journaling. Digital tools, such as audio journals and photos, can be helpful, as can conversations with trusted people. The subjects we explore will hopefully inspire you to try a variety of ways of reflecting and responding. Whatever method(s) you use will be a part of your wellness toolkit.

You will also find invitations to try strategies, explore varying perspectives, and consider new ideas aimed at well-being. Take your time with these invitations. Give yourself permission to explore. Keep in mind that you may choose to skip them at any time, depending on your personal needs. You determine your path through this book—it doesn't have to be linear. Please choose what works for you!

You might choose to read this book independently and record personal reflections. You may also want to experience the process with a colleague or small group of educators to share your learning and insights. Or this could be an opportunity for a professional learning community, shared as a grade, department, school, or even your entire school division or district. Each approach has its merits.

This book is meant to be supportive and not prescriptive. Please use it, and the ideas within it, as a resource on your journey of well-being!

Content warning: Throughout the book, our writers have shared personal stories of their struggles and learnings on their wellness journeys. Some of the stories might be difficult for some readers. We hope that you read only what feels comfortable to you.

Messages from Knowledge Keeper North Star and Elder Stan Kipling

Teaching is a highly satisfying but sometimes overwhelming profession. The stories in this book offer strategies for teachers to use for their personal wellness. These have been shared by fellow educators in the hope that other teachers can learn from their wellness journeys and perhaps apply the thinking and techniques to their own lives.

Additionally, each chapter offers valuable concepts that originate from an Indigenous worldview. These come from Elder Stanley Kipling and Knowledge Keeper North Star, who are members of Anishinaabe communities that reside in the Treaty 1 territory in what is now Manitoba. In each chapter, Elder Stan and Knowledge Keeper North Star share messages connecting Indigenous perspectives of wellness with the ideas explored in that chapter. These passages are identified by a Sacred Hoop icon.

The concepts they share suggest ways in which teachers can make deeper connections for a healthy life. In Anishinaabemowin, they call this Mino Pimatisiwin, which means "living a good life."

> "Living a good life" can mean different things to each individual. As Indigenous People, we understand each person has the right to direct their own life without interference. When we gather for healing ceremonies, we are told stories shared by Elders and Knowledge Keepers, which we call teachings.

> Yet it is understood that everyone will take a different personal meaning from each teaching and that we can only take that which we are ready for. Each time we hear a story, even if it is the same story, we may have a different understanding of the teaching than we did before.—*North Star*

It is our hope that, as you read on and each story unfolds before you, you receive what you are ready to receive and you practise what you are ready to practise. This is the approach of Mino Pimatisiwin, living a good life.

A Holistic View of Wellness

We each have our own definition of wellness, whether we have articulated it or not. One understanding of holistic health and harmony is reflected in the Sacred Hoop.

The Sacred Hoop

The Sacred Hoop is a representation of how some Indigenous Peoples view the world. It is also known by other names, such as Cosmological Circle, Circle Teachings, Hoop Teachings, Medicine Wheel, or Wheel Teachings. (Many Indigenous communities are trying to break free from using references to the Medicine Wheel and Wheel Teachings, as these are colonial terms.)

There are many different perspectives on the Sacred Hoop, depending on Nation, territory, and personal interpretations. A common theme, as represented in the Sacred Hoop by the Four Directions, is that wellness involves the whole person—their Physical, Emotional, Mental, and Spiritual selves.

When we began planning this book, Leah Fontaine shared her idea of structuring it around the Sacred Hoop teachings as a means of infusing Indigenous Knowledge throughout the book. The Sacred Hoop shown here is the one that Elder Kipling and North Star were most familiar with. It supports their thoughts and ideas and has shaped the teachings they have received throughout their lives.

> In the Sacred Hoop, the *Physical dimension* is represented by babies and children, as their physical bodies do much growing and learning when they are new to this world. The Golden Eagle sits in the East as a teacher of unconditional love for our children. The colour yellow represents the rising sun and the gift of a brand-new day. Nourishing a healthy body through exercise, nutrition, and sleep are ways to promote physical wellness.

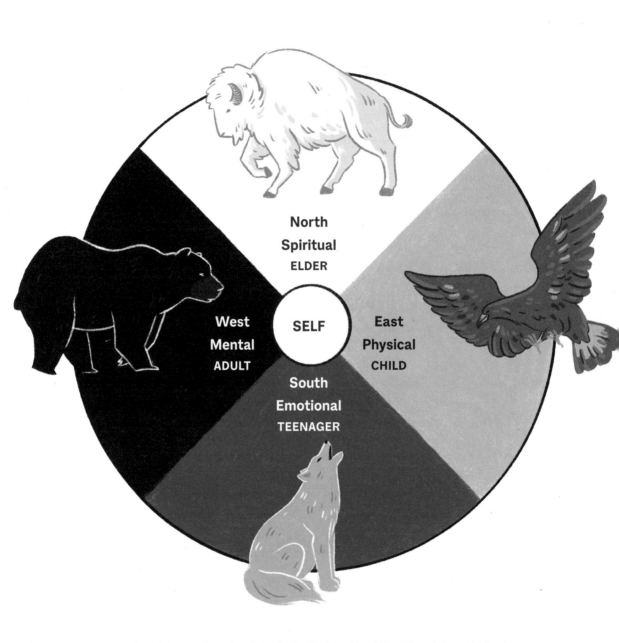

North
Spiritual
ELDER

West
Mental
ADULT

SELF

East
Physical
CHILD

South
Emotional
TEENAGER

Source: The Sacred Hoop, as shown here, is inspired by Traditional Land-Based Knowledge, which is a deep understanding of Earth and Territorial cycles that connect us to ourselves.

The *Emotional dimension* is represented by teenagers, who experience a wide range of emotions during a time of hormone changes in their lives. The Wolf sits in the South as a teacher of humility. As true leaders, wolves are humble. Although often misrepresented as wild and dangerous animals by settlers, they care for the pack even if it means their needs are not met. The colour red represents the red-hot emotions we may have during this life stage. We are teaching emotional wellness when we allow ourselves and others to experience feelings in a safe environment. Expressing emotions is a natural way to bring ourselves back into balance.

The *Mental dimension* is represented by adults, who often overthink and then worry about the decisions they have to make or the consequences of the decisions they have already made. The Black Bear sits in the West as a teacher of courage, as it takes courage to go deep within our minds and learn about patterns that no longer serve us. The colour black represents our minds and the introspection it takes to journey through our lives. Being engaged in the world through learning, problem-solving, and creativity can improve our mental wellness. Learning is an ongoing, ever-evolving, lifelong process. It keeps us forever moving and growing and prevents us from getting stuck or becoming stagnant.

The *Spiritual dimension* is represented by Elders because they have great knowledge, having travelled the path around the entire Sacred Hoop. The White Buffalo sits in the North as a teacher who teaches us about facing the toughest of challenges head-on. Because of this, both the Elders and the White Buffalo deserve much respect. The colour white represents the harsh weather we must face and the wisdom our Elders have gained, often turning their hair white in the process.

The Spiritual is that which fills us up. For some, Spirituality means connecting to our higher power, whether we call it Creator, God, Buddha, or Allah. For others, it means something different. The Spiritual also means the fire within us—our pursuits that fill us up when we feel empty. These can be dancing, singing, attending ceremonies, or painting—things that make us feel whole again. As we go deeper within ourselves, committing to another walk around the Sacred Hoop, spirituality keeps us grounded, creative, and inspired.—*North Star*

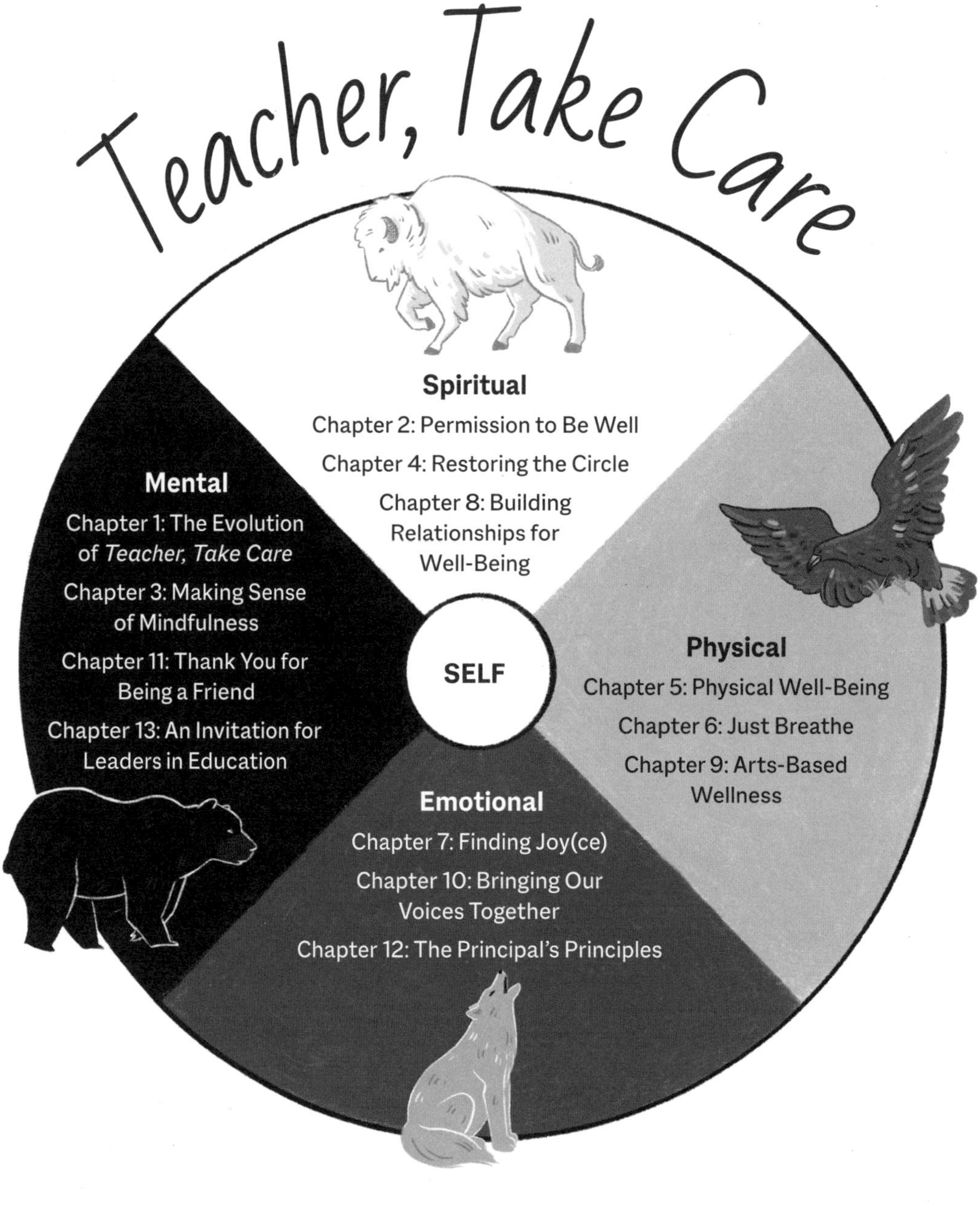

Teacher, Take Care

Spiritual

Chapter 2: Permission to Be Well

Chapter 4: Restoring the Circle

Chapter 8: Building Relationships for Well-Being

Mental

Chapter 1: The Evolution of *Teacher, Take Care*

Chapter 3: Making Sense of Mindfulness

Chapter 11: Thank You for Being a Friend

Chapter 13: An Invitation for Leaders in Education

SELF

Physical

Chapter 5: Physical Well-Being

Chapter 6: Just Breathe

Chapter 9: Arts-Based Wellness

Emotional

Chapter 7: Finding Joy(ce)

Chapter 10: Bringing Our Voices Together

Chapter 12: The Principal's Principles

Spiritual work is essential to healing. It means being on the land, talking to Mother Earth, and harvesting the gifts from the land, as when preparing hides, feathers, bones, and plants. This is spiritual medicine.—*Elder Kipling*

The framework of this book is based on the Sacred Hoop in recognition of Indigenous Knowledge and perspectives. So how does the Sacred Hoop relate to educator well-being? Taken together, the topics explored in *Teacher, Take Care* address all Four Directions. In the graphic model shown here, we have indicated where in this book you will find related materials by including the relevant chapter titles. For example, chapter 6, "Just Breathe," is linked to the Physical dimension, or East Direction. Of course, each chapter connects to the other Directions as well. Use this graphic to help you explore wellness from a holistic perspective, considering your own Physical, Emotional, Mental, and Spiritual Directions.

In using the Sacred Hoop as a framework for *Teacher, Take Care*, our purpose is also to address the Truth and Reconciliation Commission of Canada's Calls to Action, by celebrating and prioritizing Indigenous voices in the connection and transfer of knowledge, history, the legacy of Indigenous Peoples, and issues related to intercultural competency (Truth and Reconciliation Commission of Canada, 2015).

References and Further Reading

Truth and Reconciliation Commission of Canada. (2015). *Truth and Reconciliation Commission of Canada: Calls to Action*. https://nctr.ca/records/reports/#trc-reports

Chapter 1

The Evolution of Teacher, Take Care

Jennifer E. Lawson

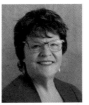

Senior author **Jennifer E. Lawson**, PhD, is the originator and program editor of the Hands-On series published by Portage & Main Press. Jennifer writes, teaches in the Faculty of Education at the University of Manitoba, and is a local school board trustee. She is also one of the founders of Mission to Mexico, an organization that supports schools in some of the most impoverished communities in Puerto Vallarta. Jennifer is a former classroom teacher, resource and special education teacher, consultant, and principal. She lives in Winnipeg, Manitoba, with her husband, Barry, and sons, Devon and Jeremy.

The year 2020 was like no other. It may have started in the usual way, at least for people living in Canada, but we were soon embroiled in a global pandemic that changed everything about our lives. This was the time that inspired the writing of *Teacher, Take Care*. However, concerns about educator wellness, or well-being (we use both terms in this book), existed long before COVID-19 and will continue to be a challenge far into the future.

Inspiration for this book came from my roles as a school trustee in Winnipeg and as an instructor in the Faculty of Education at the

University of Manitoba. In both environments, I observed first-hand the stressors affecting pre-service and practising educators. In both roles, I organized initiatives to address educator wellness, including professional development opportunities aimed at promoting resilience and fostering positive mental health. These were well received, but it was evident that much more needed to be done to support educators at the systems level to foster workplace wellness and individual well-being.

Throughout 2020, I began working with a variety of professionals in education and mental health, all of whom were passionate about supporting educators. It was during this time that the idea of a handbook on educator well-being began to evolve. Meanwhile, I was also facing my own mental health challenges. My mom, who had lived with our family, passed away at the beginning of the lockdown. Not being able to grieve together, celebrate her life with a funeral, or be supported by friends was a very difficult experience that led to a period of depression and darkness. However, this experience offered me the opportunity to re-examine my views about mental health, seek support, and begin to practise self-care.

Through my professional and personal experiences over the past few years, it has become clear that all of us, teachers included, need to take this challenging time and grow from it. And so *Teacher, Take Care: A Guide to Well-Being and Workplace Wellness for Educators* was born, offering a variety of approaches to educator self-care and well-being.

I explored many of the ideas presented in this book when addressing my own self-care. Some worked well for me, such as using the arts to foster wellness. Other approaches were more challenging. For example, mindfulness is a trial for me. What I have learned from my journey is that we need to approach self-care as individuals, respecting our sense of what helps and what doesn't.

I hope you will find something that works for you as you read through these pages.

Reflect and Respond
- In what ways was your mental health affected by the COVID-19 pandemic? What other times in your life have you found challenging?
- What strategies did you use to address your well-being?

Remember that you may respond in different ways to the prompts throughout this book. For example, you may choose to write down your thoughts, simply contemplate your responses, discuss them with a trusted friend, or express them through art or other forms of journaling.

Servant Leadership

Servant leadership is a philosophy of leading by serving based on the work of Robert Greenleaf (1991). As an educational leader, I have always been inspired by this approach and I see it as the foundation for this book. All the contributors have been practising servant leadership, as seen in their passionate commitment to the personal growth of others.

What are the characteristics of a servant-leader?

> A servant-leader is servant first. It begins with the natural feeling that one wants to serve. Then conscious choice brings one to aspire to lead. The difference manifests itself in the care taken by the servant—first, to make sure that other people's highest priority needs are being served. The best test is: do those served grow as persons; do they, while being served, become healthier, wiser, freer, more autonomous, more likely themselves to become servants? (Greenleaf, 1991, p. 7)

In essence, the servant-leader's role is to support others in a way that allows themselves and others to thrive.

As a school trustee, university instructor, and former principal, I feel that I have come closest to embodying the role of servant-leader when empowering my staff and students to succeed. Similarly, classroom teachers are servant-leaders when they are supporting students in meeting their potential. Senior school administrators can serve principals by helping to create a culture in which they can succeed and grow in their work. Principals can, in turn, create healthy environments for the staff they support. The contributors to this book, as teachers, therapists, and leaders, are together helping educators so that they can be their best physically, emotionally, mentally, and spiritually. Even within our families, we can be servant-leaders when we offer guidance and care that encourages family members to thrive.

When we support others so that they can flourish intellectually and personally, we are setting the groundwork for workplace wellness, from the individual, to the school, to the larger educational system. The visual below presents 10 characteristics of servant-leaders. These are explored in greater depth in chapter 12, "The Principal's Principles."

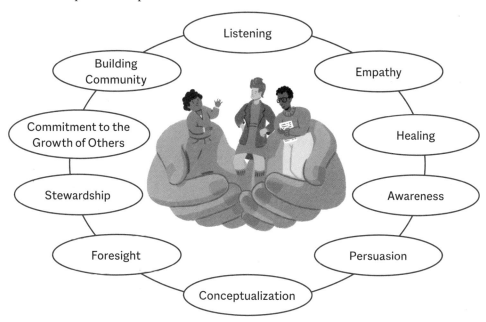

In an Anishinaabe worldview, there is something similar to the idea of a servant-leader. In our ceremonies, we have those people who help others. They prepare for ceremonies, gather wood, prepare and watch over the fire, and help our Elders do whatever needs doing. In Anishinaabemowin, this is Oshkaabewis. It is part of our Spiritual life to be of service to others. When we give back to others, we are also learning how to heal ourselves. In being of service to others, we give the best parts of ourselves.—*North Star*

Current research confirms that servant leadership can effectively support educators. It can encourage self-compassion, self-care, well-being, and well-becoming (that is, being on the journey toward wellness). Servant leadership prioritizes and promotes the needs of others, addresses emotional stress, and encourages empowerment, all of which can increase job engagement and reduce anxiety related to the workplace (Hu et al., 2020). Further, servant leadership has a positive effect on the person being served, helping to reduce emotional exhaustion, depersonalization, and burnout (Rivkin et al., 2014). Educators at all levels who embrace the role of servant-leader can help to promote psychological health and workplace wellness.

Reflect and Respond
- Consider the servant-leader traits presented on the graphic. Reflect on these traits.
- Who in your life is a servant-leader?
- How does this person foster wellness in others?

Inclusion

Diversity is a fact.
Equity is a choice.
Inclusion is an action.
Belonging is an outcome.
—*Arthur Chan*

Our team of writers understands the importance of celebrating the diversity that is reflected in our teaching and student populations. We hope that the messages we share and the approaches we take to wellness are inclusive and respectful of all. People differ in race, religion, gender, ability and disability, socioeconomic background, and more. There are differences in "how health and illness are perceived, coping styles, treatment-seeking patterns, impacts of history, racism, bias, and stereotyping, gender, family, stigma, and discrimination" (Gopalkrishnan and Babacan, 2015).

Every teacher's story is different. In sharing individual stories and exploring personal views on mental health and well-being, we have tried to reflect that diversity. Moreover, the topics in this book address equity, diversity, and inclusion issues.

When we grow to understand, appreciate, and respect the diversity around us … we gain a positive and accepting community, which benefits everyone.

This benefits individuals because when people feel accepted, respected and included, they have better mental health. When we develop the skills and attitudes that will assist us in our relationships and working life, it contributes to our collective social and emotional well-being. It also benefits organizations and communities, as environments where people enjoy positive mental health are more pro-social and more productive. (Be You, n.d.)

Understanding the issues that link equity, diversity, and mental health is a way of fostering inclusion. With this understanding, we can build a culture of well-being for all, both at the individual and the systemic level. This can have a direct, positive impact on workplace wellness.

Reflect and Respond
- Have you experienced inclusion? How did this affect your mental health?
- In what ways have you experienced exclusion? How did this affect your mental health?
- In your experience, what benefits does inclusion have on overall workplace wellness?
- What are some examples of how you foster inclusion in your workplace?

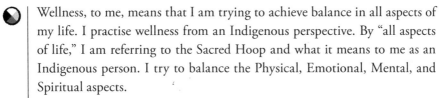

Wellness, to me, means that I am trying to achieve balance in all aspects of my life. I practise wellness from an Indigenous perspective. By "all aspects of life," I am referring to the Sacred Hoop and what it means to me as an Indigenous person. I try to balance the Physical, Emotional, Mental, and Spiritual aspects.

I encourage all people to intentionally practise an open, supportive, and caring approach when interacting with others. Try to understand where people are coming from, and work to be part of a respectful and compassionate society.—*Elder Kipling*

References and Further Reading

Be You. (n.d.). *Cultural diversity and mental health*. Retrieved May 28, 2021, from https://beyou.edu.au/fact-sheets/relationships/cultural-diversity-and-mental-health

Chan, A. (2020). *Diversity is a fact* [Post]. LinkedIn. https://www.linkedin.com/in/arthurpchan/

Crippen, C. (2005). The democratic school: First to serve, then to lead. *The Canadian Journal of Educational Administration and Policy, 47*.

Gopalkrishnan, N., & Babacan, H. (2015). Cultural diversity and mental health [Suppl.] *Australasian Psychiatry, 23*(6), 6–8. https://doi.org/10.1177/1039856215609769

Greenleaf, R. K. (1991). *The servant as leader*. Robert K. Greenleaf Center.

Hu, J., He, W., & Zhou, K. (2020). The mind, the heart, and the leader in times of crisis: How and when COVID-19-triggered mortality salience relates to state anxiety, job engagement, and prosocial behavior. *Journal of Applied Psychology, 105*(11), 1218–33. https://doi.org/10.1037/apl0000620

Rivkin, W., Diestel, S., & Schmidt, K.-H. (2014). The positive relationship between servant leadership and employees' psychological health: A multi-method approach. *German Journal of Human Resource Management, 28*(1–2). https://doi.org/10.1177/239700221402800104

Chapter 2
Permission to Be Well

Laura Doney and Dana Fulwiler Volk

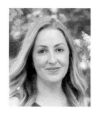 **Laura Doney**, MA, BEd, MC, is a Certified Canadian Counsellor and currently works as a therapist in Calgary, Alberta. Laura has worked in school districts for seven years in multiple roles. She completed a master of counselling degree and focused her graduate thesis on teacher mental health. Her passion for personal development and well-being is rooted in her own personal work and the belief that we are all here to learn and grow. She has presented at numerous educational conferences and conventions about the importance of personal and systemic well-being.

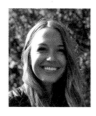 **Dana Fulwiler Volk**, BEd, MEd, MAPP, is a learner, educator, consultant, and co-founder of a well-being podcast and professional learning platform called Teacher Fan Club. Dana's experience spans public education, non-profit, and post-secondary, including roles as a classroom teacher, system leader, and instructor with the Werklund School of Education at the University of Calgary and the Positive Psychology Center at the University of Pennsylvania. Dana's current work is focused on helping individuals, workplaces, and organizational systems infuse research-informed, inclusive, and sustainable well-being practices.

Imagine it is a quiet day and you have nothing pressing that needs your attention. You decide to meet up with a new colleague to get to know each other. While you are conversing, your colleague asks you, "What's been your journey in teaching so far?" You spend time sharing stories about what brought you to the profession and about your experiences as teachers, good and bad.

What stories would you tell? Most likely, you would share only certain parts of your teaching story. In this chapter, we will guide you to reflect on the parts you tell *and* the parts you don't tell. We hope this will help you increase your awareness of the story you are living in right now and how your well-being can be influenced by your stories of teaching.

Reflect and Respond

Think about the various stories you tell yourself and others about teaching and about being well as a teacher. Here are some prompts to get you started:

- Why did you become a teacher?
- If you were to map out your journey as a teacher, how would you describe the beginning, middle, and present?
- What would be the highlights and low points of the stories you share?

You may choose to simply reflect on your answers, but we encourage you to write them down so you can return to them. Recording your story before you get very far into this book provides you with a baseline. Often, we are progressing and growing, and we don't even realize it. We hope that, by creating a record of where you started when you began this chapter, you will find it easier to see your personal growth and progress when you have finished this book.

 When helping others, I always share stories of my lived experience connected to my teachings. These stories are raw and from the heart, and the people I work with know my sharing is genuine and can feel the pain as I share.

I went into university to be an engineer, but after two years of personal reflection and seeing my classmates go through some of the same struggles

I did as a young man, I realized I could use my lived experience and my cultural practices to help others. At the time, I never thought of myself as a teacher but only as a helper.

My journey started when I wanted to heal myself by finding out why I reacted a certain way in situations and why I felt certain ways. I was unhealthy and angry at the beginning. Yet as I gained more knowledge of these behaviours and of my history, I began to understand where they were coming from. I found a history of pain and abuse, but I also found ways to deal with this trauma. I grew strong and realized how resilient I was.

The low point of my story is that, at one time, I believed that I was completely to blame for my negative feelings and behaviours. My highlights revolve around how I have used my knowledge and story to help others find a way out, grow strong, and use their experiences for good. Presently, I am only at the middle stage of my story because, as a teacher and helper, I have much to share yet.—*Elder Kipling*

The Power of Stories

We are constantly engaged in giving meaning to the experiences we have (Madigan, 2011). As we do this, themes arise and various personal narratives, or stories, are created. It can be helpful to become aware of the stories we are telling ourselves. Self-awareness is a foundation for well-being.

Throughout this book, each contributor has their personal story to tell, just as you do. Why do we believe our stories are important to include? First, they build a connection with you, the reader. Second, we want to acknowledge and validate many of the common stories we have told and heard in teaching. Third, we want to model how to reflect on your dominant story and deepen your self-awareness. And fourth, we'd like to acknowledge that we are not enlightened beings who have reached a magical destination of well-being. We struggle sometimes too, and so we do the work.

As you read Dana's story below, consider the beliefs about teaching that are embedded within it.

A Teacher's Evolving Story

When I think about my path to teaching, I go back to the feeling of holding real chalk in my hands when I played pretend. That chalk was the symbol of professionalism I longed for as an eight-year-old. I felt so empowered writing on that little blackboard in my bedroom. By the time I graduated from high school, I had shifted my career sights toward pharmacy. I had somehow learned that pharmacists make good money and are respected, and everyone assumes they are smart. At the time, those things mattered to me.

I volunteered in a pharmacy and noticed myself watching the clock, waiting to leave. I thought about that little girl with the chalk in her hand and reflected on the different ways I viewed pharmacy versus teaching. Pharmacy was clear; teaching seemed muddled. As a young person, I had heard contradictory views about the teaching profession and absorbed conflicting narratives. Teaching is an honourable calling; teaching is for people who just want summers off. Teaching is a beautiful way to inspire the next generation; teaching is for people who can't do other things. Teachers are generous and intelligent; teachers aren't actual professionals. Teachers aren't paid nearly enough; teachers are paid too much. And on and on. At that time, I valued others' approval more than my own, but my 18-year-old brain couldn't make sense of other people's opinions of teaching.

I decided to volunteer in an inner-city reading program, where I reconnected with my love of kids, learning, and education. I started to listen to my inner voice and accept that pharmacy wasn't for me. I began to share with others my desire to become a teacher. I was surprised by those who responded with warnings, even teachers themselves who recalled their own negative experiences. I also heard the exact opposite—experienced teachers saying, "It's the best thing I've ever done," or "You would make an incredible teacher!"

Eventually, I came to honour my voice and sense of purpose at the time; I became a teacher. I felt fulfilled by connections with students and colleagues and the impact I believed I was making. However, in those early years, I also felt twinges of resentment and shame. These feelings were amplified and reinforced by what I perceived as a hierarchy within the profession. For example, I rarely taught a core subject, which seemed to place me on a lower rung of the respect ladder. Over time, I developed a defensive attitude about teaching and the roles I found myself in. At times, I also felt guilt, frustration, disappointment, and loneliness.

I was looking for external validation so that I could feel proud of my role as an educator, when what I needed was to reconnect to my sense of purpose. I needed to remember my *why* and disconnect from unhelpful internalized narratives. I had to zoom out. In the process of zooming out, I was able to more clearly see the many wonderful stories that exist alongside the difficult ones. I also realized that well-being and resilience are not "do-it-yourself" endeavours.

I had the gift of starting my career in a school culture of collegiality and support. I experienced the giving and receiving of energy that happens when we feel seen, heard, and valued. Staff were encouraged to take initiative, collaborate, be authentic, and connect outside of work. Thanks to the amazing power of connection, I experienced trust, joy, and the feeling of being part of a team.

Not only did my colleagues support me as a new professional but they also supported me personally. During my first year of teaching, my Dad was diagnosed with cancer. Looking back, I see how the stress and uncertainties of a new career, living in a new city, and a parent's illness affected my relationships and well-being. I struggled to find balance. I realize now how instrumental my colleagues were to my well-being and growth. They just got it. The bonds built between us have lasted throughout the years; many of those colleagues became lifelong friends. My Dad passed away several years after I had moved on from that school, and the group card I received from them was filled with love, compassion, and meaningful stories my colleagues remembered about my Dad. It was written as if I were still part of the community.

I derived sustenance and strength from this community. I grew as an educator and a young woman through both my comfortable and uncomfortable experiences at that school. What made this school special was both our collective purpose in supporting "our kids" and the ways we prioritized fun (staff retreats, surprise air-band and dance performances, and more) and connection outside of school. We were encouraged to take risks and have vulnerable real-talk conversations that weren't always comfortable but usually resulted in growth and understanding. I felt proud to be part of this community of change-makers.

Reflect and Respond

Bring awareness to the stories you tell. Think about Dana's story. What beliefs about teaching do you see in it?

Think about the helpful or unhelpful beliefs or narratives in your own story of teaching. Return to your reflections from the beginning of this chapter and consider them through the lens of the following statements. (A few examples of possible responses are shown.) How would you fill in the blanks?

- Teaching is _____.
  (fulfilling? fun and energizing? hard and exhausting?)
- Teachers are _____.
  (superheroes? advocates? intelligent and multitalented? not as respected as other professionals?)
- As a teacher, I am _____.
- As a teacher, I am allowed to _____.
- As a teacher, I am not allowed to _____.
- Compared to other professionals, I am _____.
- My mental health as a teacher is _____.
- Well-being in teaching is _____.

What visible and hidden beliefs, ideas, and narratives are present in your responses to these statements? Be aware of and consider the beliefs that may be buried in your own story. Our stories are always forming, reforming, and evolving, inviting us to grow alongside the ebb and flow of our lives, our teaching experiences, and the lessons we learn along the way. Your story can change, and you can change your own story. Next, we will explore the process of "re-storying," beginning with some theoretical concepts.

Dominant Stories

When you tell a story about yourself as a teacher, or about teaching in general, you naturally privilege certain events over others. You focus on the experiences that fit your already established beliefs about yourself.

For example, if you think that teaching is hard, you will find examples in your experiences that support this conclusion. The more you tell stories about teaching being hard, the more solidified that belief becomes. The story of teaching being hard becomes *dominant* in your life, and you find more examples of events that fit with the meaning you have already created for other events (White, 2007). Over time, positive events that contradict this view, such as times when teaching has come more easily, become less visible. Alternately, if you think that teaching is rich and rewarding, the more you tell positive stories of teaching, the more established those beliefs become for you. These stories become dominant in your life, and the negative stories become less of a focus.

A simple visual can illustrate this concept. This is Sam. Sam has a dominant story that they are not good enough (represented by the – symbol). But of course, there are experiences where they have felt good enough and have received feedback from others that they are good enough (represented by the + symbol). However, because they believe they are not good enough, the negative experiences are easier for them to see. In other words, they subconsciously privilege those experiences. Notice how within Sam's field of vision there are way more – symbols than + symbols. This illustrates how when we focus more on the negative, we further solidify a belief in the negative. In Sam's case, this process strengthens the belief that they are not good enough.

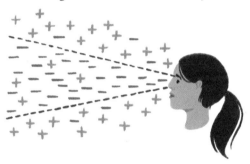

Sometimes our dominant stories are so deeply ingrained that they start to feel like the truth. But often, our descriptions of ourselves allow little space for the complexities and contradictions of life. Our built-in negativity bias further amplifies the – signs over the + signs. We are hardwired to notice and focus on the negative (Rozin and Royzman, 2001).

Can you think of a time when one negative interaction or event became all you could think about, despite several other positive events happening that very same day? We notice threats and seek problems to solve. We owe part of our survival as a species to this negativity bias (Vaish et al., 2008). However, this bias can get in the way of our well-being and ability to recognize and challenge our dominant story, thus causing us to focus on our struggles rather than our triumphs.

The meaning you give to the events you experience is not neutral in the effect it has on your life. This meaning forms and shapes your life in the future (Madigan, 2011).

For this reason, self-awareness is extremely important, as it helps us notice the stories that keep us stuck. When we are more aware of the buried and borrowed beliefs and ideas that make up our dominant narrative, we are empowered to keep them or let them go. In the following sections, we explore self-awareness strategies that can help us re-story and prioritize our well-being.

The Power of Well-Being

The Western view of well-being contains mixed messages about what's important and what to focus on. We hear about the best programs or products, the difference between well-being and wellness, and so on. The noise can be overwhelming.

One way to think of well-being is as both feeling good and functioning well (Keyes and Annas, 2009). We like this as a starting point. As you read and contemplate the ideas in this chapter, we encourage you to think deeply about the meaning of being well for you. Definitions of well-being typically vary across individuals, cultures, contexts, and even stages of life. In your early career as a teacher, for example, it may mean something different than it will 10 years in.

> **Reflect and Respond**
> To understand your own version of feeling good and functioning well, ask yourself the following questions:
> - What are the first ideas that come to mind when you think of well-being?
> - What does it mean for you to be well?
> - What daily practices in your life invite you to feel good and function well?
> - Right now, what would it mean to prioritize your well-being?

 For me, well-being is found in the Sacred Hoop, and in finding balance in the four dimensions—Physical, Emotional, Mental, and Spiritual. Well-being is essential for me because, as a teacher, I must provide others with good healing energy in everything I do and everything I say. I must practise what I preach, not only when people are watching me but also when I am alone with the Creator and Creation.

> I am Bear Clan, and the Bear teaches me and those who will listen that we must always first look within for the answers we seek. That is my inner voice. If I do not listen to my Bear voice, he will then come to me in my dreams, and that is when I know I need to slow down and take more care of myself. My wellness is connected to my own inner voice and the teachings of the Bear.—*Elder Kipling*

Positive psychology is the scientific study of what goes right in life and how to cultivate it. It's not about minimizing the real challenges that exist; it's about acknowledging and capitalizing on the real goodness that also exists. In the process, we can grow through our challenges and emerge even stronger. Positive psychology advocates for us to be just as focused on building upon what goes right with us as we are trying to alleviate what goes wrong. Even though the bad can sometimes overpower the good, we also have a capacity and desire to live life above neutral—not just to alleviate suffering or get by, but to thrive and flourish and be well.

Dr Martin Seligman is considered one of the pioneers of positive psychology. PERMA is Seligman's (2013) theory of well-being. It identifies evidence-based pathways to feeling good, functioning well, and living life above neutral. These pathways include:

- Positive emotions
- Engagement
- Relationships
- Meaning
- Accomplishment
- Health, or vitality

Although not part of Seligman's original theory, health, or vitality, is often added to PERMA by researchers and practitioners to emphasize the importance of physical nourishment to our well-being. Thus, PERMA expands to become PERMAH (McQuaid, n.d.).

The PERMAH theory has been brought into the education realm as well, as part of professional development related to workplace wellness and to supporting the well-being of students and educators. You can see from the diagram below how our well-being can be cultivated through the PERMAH pathways or building blocks.

PERMAH
Well-Being Pathways

POSITIVE EMOTIONS
Cultivating and enhancing experiences of positive emotions from the past, present, and future

HEALTH
Taking care of our bodies and minds with nourishing food and hydration, energizing and restorative movement, and quality sleep habits

ENGAGEMENT
Applying our strengths and skills in rewarding and challenging ways

ACHIEVEMENT
Experiencing a sense of accomplishment and believing in our own capacity to pursue goals and dreams

RELATIONSHIPS
Intentionally cultivating positive relationships marked by trust, authenticity, and energizing interactions

MEANING
Connecting to something larger than ourselves and feeling a sense of purpose in our lives

Reflect and Respond

What's your level of PERMAH?

The Wellbeing Lab offers a free PERMAH survey to help build your well-being awareness and explore strengths, goals, and areas for growth. It offers the option to track your progress (see <https://permahsurvey.com/>) and even suggests evidence-based practices to help you reach your well-being goals based on your results.

For more on PERMAH and how you as a leader can intentionally incorporate this model of well-being into your school culture, see chapter 12, "The Principal's Principles."

Habits Over Willpower

Taking action on well-being can be hard because behaviour change is hard. But it's still within reach! A disconnect can exist between knowing something is good for us and doing the thing that's good for us. We like rewards, but the pursuit of well-being doesn't always provide us with the instant gratification we so enjoy and crave. Willpower, once thought of as the golden key to achieving our well-being, is now considered a smaller piece of the puzzle. Research suggests that our systems and strategies—including our habits of thought and action—outperform our willpower (Wood, 2019).

Consider your history of well-being and whether your habits have leaned toward an all-or-nothing approach to well-being or more of a lifestyle-for-a-lifetime approach. Small, consistent actions that nurture our well-being are more effective than intensive but inconsistent actions. We are much more likely to sustain the slow and steady course over time.

The Role of Self-Permission and Compassion in Well-Being

> The grass is greener where you water it.
> —*Neil Barrington*

Self-permission is the way in which we allow ourselves to prioritize personal well-being and focus on a fulfilling life (Løvestam, 2019, p. 22; see also Rose, 2014). It is a psychological process that is key to the pursuit of well-being. Self-permission may include taking time to engage in enjoyable activities for their own sake, practising self-care through adequate sleep and nourishment, pursuing intrinsically motivating goals, and enjoying life without feeling guilty or apologetic (Løvestam, 2019).

Sometimes we are our own biggest barrier to pursuing well-being. We might blame external factors for why we cannot prioritize our well-being. This can be especially true for teachers, given our endless to-do lists, demands on our time, thousands of daily decisions, structured schedules, and so on. Or we might get stuck in social comparison, seeing how others seemingly manage better than us and assuming the grass is greener elsewhere. While these are certainly realities and challenges to be acknowledged, we can also look inward and ask, "Have I given myself permission to be well?"

Guilt seems to be a particularly powerful barrier to well-being and self-permission for teachers. If we're not marking, lesson planning, classroom organizing, emailing, or tending to our own family, we should be. Yet "shoulding" can lead to counter-productive, hamster-wheel thoughts—they go round and round but get us nowhere. These thoughts can cause us to miss, ignore, or misinterpret important messages in the world around us. Awareness of guilt-ridden thoughts is the beginning of changing this.

One example is when we catch ourselves getting stuck in all-or-nothing thinking: "I didn't get any of my marking done this weekend … I'm a terrible teacher and horribly unorganized … everyone must know I'm a fraud … others get their marking done faster than me." Every teacher has taken home a bag of marking and had it sit by the door all weekend, then felt guilty about it. Instead, if we can look at the bag of marking and remind ourselves that it's okay to take a self-care weekend, such positive self-talk can be comforting. We all navigate internal dialogues that can either energize or deplete us. Our unhelpful thinking patterns can have a significant impact on our overall well-being, especially in the areas of relationships and mental health (Kross, 2021). Think for a moment: When it comes to teaching, does your self-talk energize or deplete you?

Invite Self-Compassion

Self-compassion—including ourselves within the circle of care we extend to others—is one way to cultivate self-permission. As educators, we extend compassion so generously to others, yet often have a more difficult time extending it to ourselves. Directing our care inward can be a powerful way to combat self-criticism and challenge the barriers that get in the way of self-permission.

Researcher Kristin Neff (2011) explains self-compassion as treating ourselves with kindness—as we would a friend—by engaging in supportive self-talk, mindfulness practice, and approaching our situation in the context of a larger human experience. Neff's research has found that "self-compassion buffers the negative effects of suffering, meaning that people who are compassionate toward themselves are much less likely to be anxious, depressed, and stressed from the struggles of life compared to their self-critical counterparts" (MacBeth and Gumley, 2012, in Waters et al., 2021). For example, research found that participants with more self-compassion felt less traumatized by COVID-19 and had less pandemic-related anxiety (Waters et al., 2021). Learn more about Kristin Neff's research and explore free, evidence-based practices at <https://selfcompassion.org>.

Reflect and Respond
Apply this tool to build self-permission:
- When you're facing guilt about prioritizing your well-being, ask yourself, "What would I say to a friend right now?"
- Write your response to a friend for yourself and keep these words close to you.

We mentioned at the beginning of this chapter that self-awareness is foundational to well-being. The more we understand our strengths and limitations (without self-judgment), the more intentional we can be in crafting and adapting our own ideal conditions for being well. Below are 14 self-permission reflection statements adapted from a self-permission scale based on the work of Løvestam (2019) and Rose (2014). As you read them, check in with how you feel (body and mind) and the thoughts that arise when you explore concepts of self-permission. You may choose to highlight a few that resonate with you. You may want to keep these chosen statements where you can see them regularly, so they can help to ground you and set the tone for your day or to see the bigger picture in a difficult moment.

Self-Permission Statements for Reflection
1. I permit myself to pursue well-being in my life.
2. I allow myself to live a life full of meaning and purpose.
3. I deserve to flourish.
4. I let myself pursue things in life that I really cherish.
5. I allow myself to live up to my potential.
6. I deserve to be happy.
7. I let myself pursue my goals with passion.
8. I allow myself to engage in activities where I feel fully immersed in what I am doing.
9. I give myself permission to follow my aspirations.

10. I allow myself to practice self-care.
11. I permit myself to nourish my relationships and spend time with people I care about.
12. I never feel guilty for taking care of my personal well-being.
13. I let myself search for meaning in my life.
14. In general, I give myself permission to lead a good life.

What prevents you from giving yourself permission to pursue well-being? Please list one to three barriers (Løvestam, 2019, pp. 30–31).

Crafting a Story of Being Well

Our final invitation is designed to help you unearth other possible storylines, specifically your stories of practising and experiencing well-being.

We have included questions that are intended to open space for new possibilities and help you articulate stories of being well (Tomm, 1987). We hope that reflecting on these questions will make it easier for you to tell your stories of well-being, beginning here and continuing throughout this book. We encourage you to dive deeply into this activity and craft a story—your manifesto of being well—that is full of rich descriptions. This means spelling out in detail the events that make up your story of well-being. Call up memories of triumph, joy, peace, purpose, wonderment, pride, and success.

If you are deep in the habit of telling stories of being unwell, it may be difficult in the beginning for you to shift to talking about yourself as being well. (Remember our negativity bias and how we can intentionally redirect our attention by cultivating PERMAH and self-permission and compassion.) When we free up space for authentic experiences of connection and well-being in our lives, we add new layers to savour in our story. Wherever you are right now, we invite you to start there.

Reflect and Respond
Craft your story of well-being by reflecting on the following questions:
- In what ways have you already turned out to be the kind of person you dreamed of being when you were younger?

- Thinking back to a time when you felt most well as a teacher, what exactly were you doing? What was the context of your life and work at that time? What made it possible for you to take care of yourself and prioritize your well-being during past times of struggle? Which conditions could you recreate today?
- If you were to practise noticing times of triumph and contentment, more than focusing on moments of struggle and chaos, how do you imagine your inner dialogue would change? What would you be saying to yourself?
- If, instead of viewing yourself as breaking down, you shifted to viewing yourself as breaking through, how do you imagine your emotions and felt experience would shift?
- Imagine you were able to give yourself permission to be well, in whatever ways fit for you. What would this mean? What first steps would you take toward your own well-being? Who or what resources would be helpful to you in working toward this image of well-being?
- When you are deciding between caring for others or caring for yourself, how can you hold space for yourself and others at the same time, rather than having to choose?
- If you had the chance, what advice would you give to others about well-being? In what ways are you able to take your own advice now?

Source: Adapted from Tomm, 1987

Once you have finished your process of reflecting on and answering the questions above, we encourage you to continue writing your own story of being well. Use the energy from any mental and emotional shifts you may have experienced in this chapter, and as you read this book, to support you in writing your manifesto of being a "well" teacher. Whether you have committed your stories to memory or the written page, tell them to yourself, out loud and often.

I am at my best when I am doing spiritual work. I am happy, and people tell me I am glowing. Those who are more connected to the spirit say they can actually see an aura around me. I often look back on my life and say to myself, "Do you like the man you were last month, last year, 5 years or 10 years ago, or are there changes you need to make to be an even better teacher and helper?" I do not forget the struggles I had, so I can remember as I help others with similar struggles.

I have already accomplished more than what I dreamed I could be. My dreams are small in the big picture of Creation. I wanted only to go to university, get a degree, and be able to survive. I have raised a daughter on my own who has a successful career and I have been healthy enough to become a helper and teacher. I never dreamed people would value my knowledge. I have crafted a story of being well as I help others to become well.—*Elder Kipling*

Closing Thoughts

As we adventure through life, our search for well-being is a constant, fluid evolution. More important than what well-being is—and isn't—are the small actions we take each day that help us feel good and function well in a meaningful, sustainable way.

This book is filled with a menu of opportunities to use as part of your well-being practice. In exploring the stories and challenges shared here by other educators, give yourself the gift of compassion and permission to be well.

As you journey into the chapters ahead, we invite you to:

- Be open to both new ideas and to old ones that you may have previously discounted.
- Lean into new insights and opportunities, and the discomfort, vulnerability, and uncertainty that may arise.
- Start living these practices now. Remember to start small.
- Keep a record of any ideas, quotes, and "aha" moments you experience, however you choose to write your story.
- Take what works for you and leave the rest; this is about you and for you!

> Yesterday I was clever, so I wanted to change the world.
> Today I am wise, so I am changing myself.
> —*Rumi*

References and Further Reading

Brackett, M. A. (2020). *Permission to feel: The power of emotional intelligence to achieve well-being and success.* Celadon Books.

David, S. A. (2016). *Emotional agility: Get unstuck, embrace change, and thrive in work and life.* Avery.

Dulwich Centre. (n.d.). *What is narrative therapy?* Retrieved July 1, 2021, from https://dulwichcentre.com.au/what-is-narrative-therapy/

Dutton, J. E. (2003). *Energize your workplace: How to create and sustain high-quality connections at work.* Jossey-Bass.

Dutton, J. E., & Heaphy, E. D. (2003). The power of high-quality connections. In K. S. Cameron, J. E. Dutton, & R. E. Quinn, (Eds.), *Positive organizational scholarship: Foundations of a new discipline* (pp. 263–78). Berrett-Koehler Publishers.

Fredrickson, B. L. (2001). The role of positive emotions in positive psychology: The broaden-and-build theory of positive emotions. *American Psychologist, 56*(3), 218–26. https://www.ncbi.nlm.nih.gov/pmc/articles/PMC3122271/

Jiménez, Ó., Sánchez-Sánchez, L. C., & García-Montes, J. M. (2020). Psychological impact of COVID-19 confinement and its relationship with meditation. *International Journal of Environmental Research and Public Health, 17*(18), 6642.

Keyes, C. L. M., & Annas, J. (2009). Feeling good and functioning well: Distinctive concepts in ancient philosophy and contemporary science. *The Journal of Positive Psychology, 4*(3), 197–201. doi:10.1080/17439760902844228

Kross, E. (2021). *Chatter: The voice in our head, why it matters, and how to harness it.* Crown.

Løvestam, C. L. (2019*). Self-permission and well-being: Self-permission as a "key" to flourishing in therapy and positive interventions.* (Publication Number 164) [Master of Applied Positive Psychology (MAPP) Capstone Project, University of Pennsylvania]. Scholarly Commons. https://repository.upenn.edu/cgi/viewcontent.cgi?article=1167&context=mapp_capstone

Madigan, S. (2011). *Narrative therapy.* Washington, DC: American Psychological Association.

McQuaid, M. (n.d.). *What is PERMAH?* Retrieved July 1, 2021, from https://permahsurvey.com/the-science/

Neff, K. (2011). *Self-compassion: The proven power of being kind to yourself.* William Morrow.

Rose, N. (2014). *Introducing self-permission: Theoretical framework and proposed assessment.* (Publication Number 59) [Master of Applied Positive Psychology (MAPP) Capstone Project, University of Pennsylvania]. Scholarly Commons. https://repository.upenn.edu/cgi/viewcontent.cgi?article=1059&context=mapp_capstone

Rozin, P., & Royzman, E. B. (2001). Negativity bias, negativity dominance, and contagion. *Personality and Social Psychology Review, 5*(4), 296–320. https://doi.org/10.1207/S15327957PSPR0504_2

Seligman, M. E. P. (2013). *Flourish: A visionary new understanding of happiness and well-being.* Atria.

Tomm, K. (1987). Interventive interviewing: Part II. Reflexive questioning as a means to enable self-healing. *Family Process, 26*(2), 167–83. doi:10.1111/j.1545-5300.1987.00167.x

Tomm, K., St. George, S., Wulff, D., & Strong, T. (2014). *Patterns in interpersonal interactions: Inviting relational understandings for therapeutic change.* Routledge.

Vaish, A., Grossmann, T., & Woodward, A. (2008). Not all emotions are created equal: The negativity bias in social-emotional development. *Psychological Bulletin, 134*(3), 383–403. doi:10.1037/0033-2909.134.3.383

Waters, L., Algoe, S. B., Dutton, J., Emmons, R., Fredrickson, B. L., Heaphy, E., Moskowitz, J. T., Neff, K., Niemiec, R., Pury, C., & Steger, M. (2021). Positive psychology in a pandemic: Buffering, bolstering, and building mental health. *The Journal of Positive Psychology, 17*(3), 303–23. doi:10.1080/17439760.2021.1871945

White, M. (2007). *Maps of narrative practice.* W. W. Norton.

Wood, W. (2019). *Good habits, bad habits: The science of making positive changes that stick.* Farrar, Straus, and Giroux.

Chapter 3

Making Sense of Mindfulness

Keith Macpherson

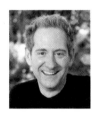

Keith Macpherson, BEd, author, speaker, and certified professional co-active life coach through the Co-Active Training Institute, is a global leader in improving overall mental health and wellness. In his bestselling book, *Making Sense of Mindfulness*, Keith introduces his five-step framework for practically integrating this powerful practice into daily life. Keith is also known for his work as a professional musician, most notably being a top finalist on the hit television series *Canadian Idol.* Keith is active on social media and inspires thousands of people around the world with his "daily intentions."

Several years ago, I was teaching yoga classes at a local studio in my hometown of Winnipeg, Manitoba. After one class, a student approached me with an invitation to lead a professional development session for a group of educators on the topic of mindfulness. With barely a thought, I jumped at the golden opportunity to volunteer. I was so ready to expand my horizons as a yoga instructor and developing keynote speaker, and this seemed like my perfect chance.

On the day of the session, I stood at the front of the classroom, gazing out into a room full of intelligent and dedicated educators who were all ready to learn about this movement of mindfulness. From me.

They looked straight at me, interested, prepared to be enlightened by my deep inner knowledge and experience with the topic. I could feel the energy of their collective anticipation of what I was about to say. I could sense my quickening heart, my damp palms. I could hear the silence of the words I wasn't yet speaking. I could see their searching eyes, peering into mine, asking what was taking me so long to start talking.

Well, I had a problem. Even though I had prepared for this workshop, I realized, at that moment, that I was not the expert that I thought I was. I did know that mindfulness was a recent buzzword in the yoga community and that I was practising it myself, but I had probably agreed too quickly to do this professional development session. And I hadn't considered that I would be teaching teachers, who have a hidden gift of knowing how to spot cheaters.

To open the dialogue and engage the group, I decided to go around the room and ask participants what mindfulness meant to them.

One teacher said, "Mindfulness, isn't that the practice where everyone sits in a circle and is given a raisin to smell, feel, and taste?"

Another replied, "Isn't that where you sit on a meditation cushion and do nothing?"

Another response was, "I have a mindfulness practice that I have on my to-do list as a morning routine. It gets me ready for the day ahead."

The conversation continued with us sharing ideas, practising strategies, and building a common understanding of mindfulness. But by the end of the session, I had many more questions than answers. I bet the teachers felt much the same way. This was the real-life experience that sent me on a fabulous journey to demystify the buzzword mindfulness. Years later, I looked back and realized that, in naively saying yes to an opportunity, I had embarked upon a lifelong journey that would change my life.

Now, I'm going to do what I did in that session years ago. Please take a moment and ask yourself the following question.

Reflect and Respond
What does mindfulness mean to you?

I hope that by the end of the chapter, you will have found some new awareness about this practice and come up with some ideas for how you can integrate it into your daily life. Or perhaps, if you have already incorporated mindfulness into your routine of well-being, you will build on your current practice.

The History of Mindfulness

The principles of mindfulness involve, in essence, "paying attention to what is happening moment by moment in a relaxed way" (Nicolai, 2020, p. xiii).

The practice of mindfulness originated in various traditions and has both religious and secular roots. Hinduism and Buddhism have been deeply influential in its evolution, and the practice of yoga has inspired much of the current attention to this practice. More recently, non-religious meditation, including the Mindfulness-Based Stress Reduction Program founded by Jon Kabat-Zinn (n.d.), has also played a part. In my research, I have learned that many Indigenous cultures also have practices embedded into their traditions that contribute to present-day understandings of mindfulness.

 Indigenous mindfulness is a practice that integrates seamlessly with all aspects of everyday life. Throughout the day, while our bodies are moving, we are being mindful of ourselves and our surroundings. Quiet prayer and gratitude is something that happens all the time.—*North Star*

The Benefits of Mindfulness

Regular mindfulness practice has many positive benefits. Research continues to show the major role that mindfulness plays in increasing our overall mental health. Here are a few of the key benefits that can occur as a direct result of integrating this practice into your daily life:

Mindfulness reduces stress. Mindfulness practice significantly decreases anxiety, depression, and somatic distress (Farb et al., 2010).

Mindfulness increases resilience. Mindfulness can increase resilience in the face of difficult emotions. The practice is also thought to enhance cognitive processes such as focus and memory. Researchers have found that "individuals with higher mindfulness have greater resilience, thereby increasing their life satisfaction." Further, those who are more mindful "can better cope with difficult thoughts and emotions without becoming overwhelmed or shutting down" emotionally (Bajaj and Pande, 2016, p. 64).

Mindfulness prevents burnout. Practising mindfulness can promote well-being, lower levels of frustration, and even act as protection against the challenges of a difficult work environment (Schultz et al., 2015).

Further research suggests that mindfulness also improves mental stamina, increases working memory, improves creativity, and increases attention and focus. It also builds emotional intelligence, which is our ability to handle our emotions and those of others (Jha et al., 2007).

Practising Mindfulness

There are many ways to incorporate mindfulness into your daily life. Many mindfulness practices refer to the following three elements: mindful breathing, mindfulness of emotions, and mindfulness of everyday life.

Mindful breathing: Bring conscious awareness to your breath in the present moment. By becoming aware of your breathing in the present moment, you may experience an instant calming effect on the nervous system and an increased degree of present-moment attention. Or you may prefer other mindfulness practices.

Mindfulness of emotions: Become aware of the emotions and feelings that you are experiencing in the present moment. You may experience clarity and deeper awareness, which can assist you in navigating forward in a calm and clear state.

Mindfulness of everyday life: Presence is power. Becoming mindful of moments where you can be fully present allows you to completely soak them in. Because your mind cannot be in two places at once, this helps you to stop overthinking (or ruminating), so you can focus your experience on where you are now. It can also help you to know where to place attention, as energy flows where attention goes (Robbins, n.d.). In addition, mindfulness in everyday life reminds you that everything that crosses your path has important messages to share. When you slow down and pay attention in the present moment, you will realize that everything you need is taking place here and now.

Practise Now: Grounding

A great place to start practising mindfulness is with the skill of grounding.

To get present in the moment, try this:

- Place your feet on the floor and become aware of the bottoms of your feet (or shoes) touching the ground in this moment.
- Feel the bottoms of your feet connecting to the ground and become aware of the sensations you notice in your feet. Perhaps they are buzzing or tingling, grounded, warm, cold, heavy, or light?
- Whatever you notice, slow down, and just spend the next few moments being present to the experience of your feet on the floor.

Once you feel grounded, focused, and aware of this moment, return to this chapter with a newfound sense of presence. Continue reading with the same practice of mindful awareness.

 One of many ceremonies that grounds and ties the Anishinaabe People to the land is our Walking-Out Ceremony. When babies are born, they are carried either in the arms of a loved one or on a tikinagan, which in English is a cradleboard. Our children are not put on the ground, touching flesh to Earth, for 13 months (one calendar year for us here in Treaty 1 territory), until they are ready to walk on their own. When that day arrives, the community gathers to witness and celebrate this special event. Barefoot, the child is placed by its parents on the Earth for the first time. This ceremony cements the relationship between the child and the Earth, creating a profound bond, so the child will respect and protect the territory they live in.—*North Star*

How Are You Being?

Mindfulness can be more than an item on your to-do list. It can be a practice of noticing *how you are being* while you are doing everything else on your to-do list. Mindfulness is all about paying attention in the present moment while being kind to yourself, other people, and the world around you.

Practise Now: Being

By becoming present with your state of being while you are reading this chapter, you are practising mindfulness.

Reflect and Respond

Right now, in this moment, take at least three deep breaths and observe yourself. Ask yourself these questions and notice what you discover.

- How am I being in this moment while I am reading this chapter?
- Is my mind racing around with distracting thoughts?
- Am I feeling connected to the words I am reading?
- What am I emotionally feeling right now? Am I joyful? Happy? Sad? Frustrated? Neutral?
- What do I notice about the state of my being in this moment?

When you become aware of how you are being while you are doing the various activities in your life (in this instance, reading), you gain insight into what is taking place under the surface of your actions. You become more aware of your feelings and emotions, your motivations, your distractions, and your intentions in each moment.

By increasing your self-awareness, you can better navigate the busyness all around you. In each moment you can make more conscious choices about where you can most effectively focus your attention.

Why Being Present?

It sounds simple to pay attention in the present moment, but consider how often we are not present in the moment at hand. For many of us, we are thinking about the parent that we had to deal with this morning over the phone, the lesson plan that still needs to be fine-tuned, or the students in our class who are struggling. Perhaps we are thinking of all the pressure and demands from above. Or maybe we are wondering how we are going to fit in grocery shopping after work along with a workout at the gym, plus getting our kids to soccer practice on time.

In one recent study, it was determined that the average human mind wanders approximately 47 percent of the time (Killingsworth and Gilbert, 2010). When technology distracts us and targeted advertising sends us messages that suggest we must do more, be more, and acquire more so that we don't miss out, it is even more challenging to be mindfully present. Recent research shows that technology is directly linked to higher levels of mind-wandering.

Do you know what this potentially means? According to these statistics, you will only be reading half of this chapter. You will have to read it a second time to get the full story. You are missing out on approximately half of your life in the present moment!

The truth is, being present is a rarity in our lives. Instead, our mind pulls us in and out of past and future thoughts. This flitting from thought to thought can wreak havoc on our nervous system and lead to increased stress and anxiety.

It is not always necessary to be present in the moment. In fact, sometimes we must wander outside the moment in our imagination to plan for upcoming events or review a past situation. When we drift out of the present moment, however, oftentimes our conditioned mind-story is focused on thoughts of fear, worry, doubt, and anxiety. In these moments, we must train ourselves to notice our current condition and make an effort to return to the present moment.

Anchoring

Many people want to be more present so that they can enjoy more moments in their life. You may be curious about how to do this. One of the most effective ways to formally train our minds to return to the present moment, especially when our mind wanders out of control, is through a popular mindfulness practice known as anchoring. Anchoring is exactly what it sounds like. You use a consistent focal point to anchor your attention to the present moment and try to keep your attention there for a designated period. When your mind wanders from the focal point (which it most likely will), you simply notice that your attention has drifted away from the anchor point, and then gently return your attention back to the anchor.

 Anchoring is like the Sundance teaching for those Indigenous Peoples who practise the Sundance Ceremony. When we are Sundancing, we are asked to shut out the busyness of daily life. It is in the Sundance circle that our spirit is finding its balance in ceremony. As Sundancers, we focus our attention on dancing, on the drumming and singing, and on the centre tree, called the Tree of Life.—*North Star*

Studies show that people who regularly practise anchoring their attention in the present moment through mindfulness are more focused, calm, and effective at each task they perform as they journey through the day (Davis and Hayes, 2012).

Anchoring does not have to be a separate formal practice during your day, especially if you don't have the time to commit to it daily. You can integrate an anchoring practice into almost every task you perform. From the conversations you are having with other people, to tasting each bite of the meal you are eating, to the two-minute task of brushing your teeth, an anchoring practice invites you to bring your full attention to the present moment or task at hand. You may find deeper connection in your conversations, better-tasting food, and maybe even fewer trips to the dentist's office. These are all examples of mindfulness in everyday life.

Practise Now: Anchoring

You may choose to practise anchoring by using a visual anchor, such as a glass of water, a candle flame, a flower, a tree, or any object that remains constant in the present moment. When your attention gets pulled away, bring yourself back to focusing on the anchor. Or you may prefer to use a tangible object that you can touch for anchoring—gently clasping a smooth stone, petting an animal, or running your hand over a soft blanket.

When you use an object as an anchor, you gently rest your attention on the object. Whenever you notice that your mind has wandered, you acknowledge that and gently return your attention to the present moment.

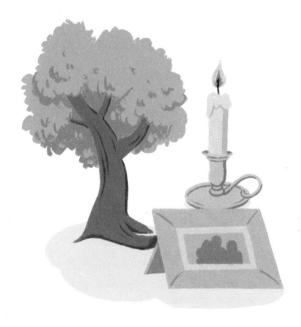

Another option, which I prefer, is to close your eyes and place your full attention on your breathing. Become aware of your inhaled breath entering your nose and your exhaled breath spilling out through your nose or mouth. Keep your attention on each segment of your breath, and when your thoughts drift and you become distracted, without any self-judgment, return to observing your breath.

I recommend setting an alarm to time your practice. You may choose to begin with a minute and work your way up to 20 minutes or longer. When you notice you have become distracted, anchor back to your object or breath. If you find that you are better able to form a routine of practice for 5 minutes at a time, you will still benefit. Even short practices can have a positive effect on the entire body (Halliwell, 2020).

Next time you catch yourself in worry mode, take a deep breath and come back to the present moment by choosing to anchor. *Now* is the moment of power.

Would you like to practise anchoring? Try these resources:
- <https://www.keithmacpherson.ca/>
- Apps such as Calm, Headspace, Aura, Insight Timer, Omnava, Stop Breathe Think, and Ten Percent Happier. (Several of these apps include meditations for parents and children.)

When We Are Truly Present, There Is No FEAR

When we are fully present in our lives, we gain clarity and become more effective at whatever task we are performing. At the same time, we lower our anxiety levels. We release our worries and fears about a future that is still yet to come and a past that has already taken place.

When you are truly present in the moment, there is no FEAR!

FEAR, in the mindfulness framework, is an acronym for False Evidence Appearing Real. Have you ever noticed that most of what you worry about in the present moment doesn't happen? Our fearful mind-stories can pull us into a future that seems so real but has not happened yet.

In a recent study, participants were asked to write down their specific worries. Then they were tracked for 30 days. By the end of those 30 days, 91 percent of the participants' feared outcomes ended up not taking place. And even when the remaining 9 percent of worries did come to pass, the result was better than expected about a third of the time (Gillihan, 2019).

Five hundred years ago, philosopher Michel de Montaigne said, "My life has been filled with terrible misfortune; most of which never happened" (de Montaigne, 1877). Can you imagine how much time and energy would be saved, and how much more inner peace would be cultivated, if we mindfully stopped ourselves from worrying about the worst-case scenarios and instead anchored in the present moment?

Everything Begins as an Inner Dream

One of the key principles of mindfulness practice is that everything begins as an inner dream. The thoughts we choose to think are like seeds being planted in the garden of our inner imagination. Over time, these thoughts eventually show up in the world around us.

Take a moment right now to look around and notice that anything you focus your attention on was once only imagined. From the clothes you are wearing to the seat you may be sitting on, many things in this physical world were once only a thought in someone's imagination.

The following exercise is a simple mindfulness practice for inner dreaming.

Reflect and Respond

What's your dream?

- Make a list of at least five different dreams you currently hold for yourself. (For example, perhaps you want to become a school administrator, complete your master's degree, or teach abroad. Or you want to learn to play the banjo or hike a famous trail.)
- Once you have declared five dreams, for each one, list at least three thoughts that you can think regularly to move in the direction of these dreams. As an example, for completing a graduate degree:
  1. The right opportunity is waiting for me right now!
  2. I can do this!
  3. One step at a time, one course at a time!

As you can see, positive thoughts can help pave the way to making dreams come true.

When you become aware of your inner dreams and use your present-moment thinking to consciously support what you are desiring, you are practising mindfulness. This is a powerful way to set your intentions and can help you to move toward your inner dreams.

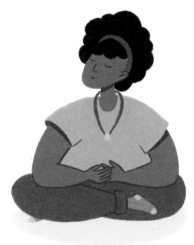

Many Indigenous Peoples, since time immemorial, have deeply understood dreams and visions as part of our daily lives. When Fasting and Vision Questing, we ground ourselves to the land and remain present while also having dreams and visions that guide us toward our future. This is, of course, a beautiful way for our Ancestors to give us guidance about our roles and responsibilities within our communities.—*North Star*

Perspective

What types of thoughts do you regularly think? Do your thoughts build you up or are they beating you up? For many of us, we gravitate toward repetitive thoughts that beat us up. (You can read about negativity bias in chapter 2, "Permission to Be Well.")

Research has shown that the average human thinks up to 60,000 thoughts per day. According to one large-scale study, 80 percent of those thousands of thoughts were negative and 95 percent were the same repetitive thoughts as the day before (Antanaityte, n.d.). This creates a negative perspective, which works against our well-being in many ways. It can lead to sabotaging the dreams that we have for ourselves. However, when we are consistently thinking thoughts that support the dream we wish to be living, we rise up, and our mental health benefits.

Yet in many of our conversations, in the staff room at lunch or at the dinner table at home, we dwell on stories of gossip, drama, negativity, and fear. It is no surprise that this has become a common practice for many people. Thoughts of fear and negativity are broadcast as breaking news stories and through constant social media feeds. In a world that has been conditioned to focus on fear and negativity, it can be easy to absorb this negative thinking and pass it on to others. Even when we want to work in a healthier school climate, we can unconsciously contribute to negativity within our teams. Being mindful of our emotions while also embracing positive thoughts and conversations is a great way to model and support a culture of workplace wellness.

A mindfulness practice invites you to become aware of your perspective and consciously assert your authority. Often, we unconsciously give away our authority to the outside world, allowing someone else to decide how we will experience our world. Consider that the word "authority," when broken down, actually contains the word "author." You can be the author of your life.

Reflect and Respond
- Who is the author of your life? Who has authority over your life?
- What is the dream you hold for yourself for your well-being?
- How do you want to feel as an educator, both in and outside of the classroom and school?

 Teachers need to be aware that the Indigenous children we encounter, as residential school intergenerational Survivors and inheritors of trauma, may still suffer the impact of these colonial legacies. They represent another form of authority, in which Indigenous Peoples were not and are not authors of their own lives. I often talk to my students about the negative voice inside my head and how I purposefully engage myself in activities that change my narrative to a positive one. For many of us, we have to actively pursue a positive voice inside our heads, replacing the negative one that was intentionally given to us to destroy us. This enables us to be empowered and to be authors of our own lives.—*North Star*

How do you become the authority—or author—of your life? When you mindfully become aware of the thoughts you are usually thinking. When you practise choosing to think and speak out loud only those thoughts that align with what you want to experience. You can live more consciously and powerfully, refining your perspective and outlook on life, when you are the author of the story you regularly choose to tell yourself.

This idea relates to the concept of re-storying, introduced in chapter 2, "Permission to Be Well." Look back at the image (on page 31), which shows the many negative thoughts we may see in our own story. Remember that we can use skills and strategies to focus more on positive thoughts and improve our overall well-being.

Practise Now: Perspective
Become aware of how your perspective influences your outlook and actions. This is an important step in living more powerfully.

Reflect and Respond
I invite you to complete each of the statements below as if in a regular conversation. Do this now, without overthinking it, and be honest with yourself.

- Work is _____.
- Time is _____.
- Money is _____.
- My students are _____.
- My to-do list is _____.
- My personal life is _____.
- This book is _____.
- I am _____.

Notice what comes up. Are there any surprises?

The way you chose to complete each statement (or any sentence, for that matter) is based on your current beliefs and the story that you have been telling yourself about that subject. Do these stories match whatever it is that you are desiring in your life? If not, you can make a mindful choice to change it, beginning right now.

If you want to make a mindful shift in what you choose to believe about something or someone, then first you must create a new story in your mind. Repeat the new story to yourself often. For example, you might begin with messages showing intention and progress, such as, "I am getting better at finishing everything on time and in a better way." Eventually, you may move toward, "Time is always available to me, and I will complete everything I desire at the right time and in the right way."

When you first tell a new story, you may experience some resistance, especially if the previous story was one that you have been thinking about and sharing for a long time. Neuroscientist Dr Rick Hanson (2009) explains that we are Velcro to negativity and Teflon to positivity. This means you need not only to have patience with yourself; you also need to practise.

To complete a mindful shift in your beliefs, you must begin emotionally programming yourself to feel the new story to be true. For example, in my new belief, "Time is always available to me, and I will complete everything I desire at the perfect time and in the perfect way," I close my eyes and imagine what it will feel like when this becomes reality.

I imagine my schedule is clearer and I am not frantically racing around from one event to the next. I assume the feeling of this new story is taking place in my emotional body as if it has already taken place. I feel my breath deepen and my chest relax. The more I think and feel this new story to be true, the sooner I will begin to experience this in my outer world.

Closing Thoughts

As author and teacher Wayne Dyer states, "When you change the way you look at things, the things you look at change" (Dyer, 2009). When we mindfully practise being present, we become more consciously aware of what we are thinking and dreaming and can begin to create the world that we wish to live in.

Now...

Breathe in, breathe out. Notice your breath.

Feel your feet on the ground.

Notice how you are feeling in this moment, without judgment.

Remember the story you are holding for yourself.

Breathe again.

Now, look at the world around you, knowing you can dream in it.

References and Further Reading

Antanaityte, N. (n.d.). *Mind matters: How to effortlessly have more positive thoughts.* TLEX Institute. Retrieved September 1, 2021, from https://tlexinstitute.com/how-to-effortlessly-have-more-positive-thoughts/

Backarova, M. (2016). The intersection between technology, mind-wandering, and empathy. In S. Y. Tettegah & D. L. Espelage (Eds.), *Emotions, technology, and behaviors* (pp. 47–62). Elsevier Academic Press.

Bajaj, B., & Pande, N. (2016). Mediating role of resilience in the impact of mindfulness on life satisfaction and affect as indices of subjective well-being. *Personality and Individual Differences, 93,* 63–67. https://doi.org/10.1016/j.paid.2015.09.005

Davis, D., & Hayes, J. (2012, July/August). What are the benefits of mindfulness? *Monitor on Psychology, 43*(7), 64. https://www.apa.org/monitor/2012/07-08/ce-corner

Dyer, W. (2007). *Change your thoughts, change your life: Living the wisdom of the Tao.* Hay House.

———. (2009). Success secrets. *Dr. Wayne W. Dyer.* https://www.drwaynedyer.com/blog/success-secrets/

Farb, N. A. S., Anderson, A. K., Mayberg, H., Bean, J., McKeon, D., & Segal, Z. V. (2010). Minding one's emotions: Mindfulness training alters the neural expression of sadness. *Emotion, 10*(1), 25–33. https://doi.org/10.1037/a0017151

Gillihan, S. (2019, July 19). How often do your worries actually come true? *Psychology Today.* https://www.psychologytoday.com/us/blog/think-act-be/201907/how-often-do-your-worries-actually-come-true

Halliwell, E. (2020, January 7). Why mindfulness meditation begins with the breath. https://www.mindful.org/6-reasons-why-mindfulness-begins-with-the-breath/

Hanson, R. (2009). *Take in the good.* https://www.rickhanson.net/take-in-the-good/

Jha, A. P., Krompinger, J., & Baime, M. J. (2007). Mindfulness training modifies subsystems of attention. *Cognitive, Affective, and Behavioral Neuroscience, 7*(2), 109–19. https://doi.org/10.3758/CABN.7.2.109

Kabat-Zinn, J. (n.d.) *Guided mindfulness meditation practices with Jon Kabat-Zinn.* Mindfulnesscds.com. Retrieved September 1, 2021, from https://www.mindfulnesscds.com/

Killingsworth, M. A., & Gilbert, D. T. (2010, November). A wandering mind is an unhappy mind. *Science, 330*(6006), 932. https://www.science.org/doi/10.1126/science.1192439

Macpherson, K. (2018). *Making sense of mindfulness.* Morgan James.

———. (n.d.) *Keith Macpherson.* Retrieved September 1, 2021, from www.keithmacpherson.ca

de Montaigne, M. (2016 [1877]). *Essays of Michel de Montaigne* (C. Cotton, Trans.; W. C. Hazlitt, Ed.). https://www.gutenberg.org/files/3600/3600-h/3600-h.htm

Nicolai, K. (2020). *Nothing much happens: Calming stories to soothe your mind and help you sleep.* Penguin Random House.

Robbins, T. (n.d.) *Where focus goes, energy flows.* Retrieved July 19, 2022, from www.tonyrobbins.com

Schultz, P., Ryan, R., Niemiec, C., Legate, N., & Williams, G. (2015, September). Mindfulness, work climate, and psychological need satisfaction in employee well-being. *Mindfulness, 6*(5), 971–85. https://doi.org/10.1007/s12671-014-0338-7

Chapter 4

Restoring the Circle
One Indigenous Perspective on Wellness
Lisa Dumas Neufeld

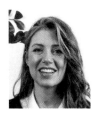

Lisa Dumas Neufeld is a Métis-Mennonite educator from Winnipeg, Manitoba. She currently teaches in an alternative high school, at an adult education centre, and in the Faculty of Education at the University of Winnipeg. She is a mother, a writer, and a local-national-international speaker. Lisa uses her personal and professional experiences to serve and share in the areas of Indigenous education, trauma, addiction and recovery, transformation, and reconciliation.

There must have been a time, way back, when my father's family was well and their Sacred Circles overflowed with light and joy and wholeness. But by the time I got here, alongside the resilience and beauty they embodied, there was unprocessed inter-generational trauma that had ravaged and wrecked them—leading to mental illness, poverty, physical disease, addiction, and abuse. Still, I know in my bones that there was a time when health, harmony, and Métis pride reigned, a time when their Circles were full and fruitful. (I use the term Sacred Circle in this chapter, which is synonymous with the Sacred Hoop.)

By the time I was a teenager, I had followed in certain familial footsteps and found myself disconnected, ill, and destructive. I was living a transient life, shuffling from foster home to group home with my belongings in garbage bags and my dignity discarded. I was unwell in every way. My Circle was fragmented. I had dropped out of school several times and was hunting for comfort wherever I could find it. My world, internally and externally, was fraught with turbulence. I became a young mother. I was unrooted, unstable, and focused mostly on survival. I was living within what I call the Realm of Risk: where a high-risk individual is so embedded within a subculture of risk that it becomes the norm (Neufeld, 2022, p. 2).

Walking out of that lifestyle has been a two-decade journey for me. With the support of many mentors, and by making some tough, positive decisions, I was able to change the trajectory of my life, "little by slow." I will share details of my journey throughout this chapter, but the short story is that I eventually went back to school and became a teacher. I now work with young adults, many of whom are dealing with the same challenges that I experienced in my early life. Still, the quest for wellness is far from complete. I've slowly been moving toward naming, reclaiming, and healing. I've been walking toward an inner reconciliation and a deep restoration. I would like to share the story of how I healed and the ways I have been able to help others do the same for themselves.

My people come from The Pas, by way of the Red River Settlement and St Laurent. I am a descendant of the Ducharme, Lavallee, and Roulette families from St Laurent, and the Dumas family from The Pas. I grew up in Winnipeg and only learned I was Métis when I was in university. As I grew up, my father was absent. My mother would share bits of stories that she'd heard from him. I'm still trying to gather up the pieces, dust them off, and put them together. I've learned that my family was a very musical, resilient group of people. Yet their culture was blunted by trauma and racism. As a young boy, my father witnessed his father's death by suicide. I can't imagine what it was like for him, his siblings, and my grandmother in a shattered Circle. My grandmother's untreated mental health issues were amplified as she tried to learn English and raise her nine surviving children alone. Two of her eleven children had passed away before her husband died.

Around this time, my father was sent to Sacred Heart, the Roman Catholic day school in The Pas. Day schools for First Nations people were part of the Canadian government's Indigenous assimilation policy. However, because it wasn't clear which level of government was responsible for educational funding for my people, as we were without a treaty, many Métis day schools were run by religious institutions with only some government involvement. These schools were operated by many of the same groups that ran the residential schools. Although my father and other Métis did not live at the schools, they suffered from many of the same traumas as residential school Survivors, including physical, emotional, sexual, and cultural abuse. My father would share stories with my mom about the abuse that he suffered at the hands of priests and nuns because of his heritage. At the time, if you could pass as French Canadian, you did.

So, while ideally, "the shared history of a people is remembered and passed on to future generations" (Macdougall, 2017, p. 27), that wasn't a reality for my family. There was a lot of secrecy and confusion about my family's history and identity, so I have experienced some serious insecurity about this. I share this story hoping that it helps another struggling person courageously begin to gather the pieces of their own identity. There have been times when I didn't feel "Métis enough" or felt that I didn't fit anywhere. There have been other times when I'd sit full of goosebumps and tears, listening to an Elder's hushed prayer, not intellectually understanding the words said, but physically-spiritually—in my bones—understanding something deep and whole and well.

When I first saw the word *pakiiwew* in an online Michif dictionary, tears streamed down my face. Pakiiwew means "to return home." My perspective is that of an urban Métis woman, once disconnected from healthy community, now finding her way back home. My stories and teachings were not gathered over cups of tea with aunties or while walking along the creek with grandparents. They come from a variety of people who showed up along my path, and I'm beyond grateful. I gathered the teachings like berries, learning from a lovely Anishinaabe grandmother and from neighbours, friends, and students of all ages. I've learned from students' parents and from colleagues, from people in recovery rooms, from speakers such as North Star and Gramma Shingoose, and leaders such as Leah Gazan and Métis Elder Barbara Bruce. I've also been blessed and nourished by Elders and Knowledge Keepers who have shared their stories and teachings through writing and film.

My thankfulness for the helpers and teachers who have shown up along my path is immeasurable. You've given me life.

Many of the teachings I've received were not directly related to the Métis culture, and at times I have felt "less than" because of that. Yet I've come to see that this feeling is also a stark post-colonial reality. I share this vulnerability knowing I'm not alone. Several of my university students have shared their recent discovery and confusion regarding their Métis-ness and their thirst for roots and teachings. Perhaps this post-colonial weaving of stories and ways is like a Métis sash: different threads are integrated into something good and complicated, something bold, useful, and sacred.

This chapter represents one evolving Indigenous perspective on wellness. Given the diversity of Indigenous cultures and experiences, we must acknowledge the danger of a single story (Adichie, 2009). Like the diversity of plants and creatures in a forest, there are many stories and perspectives among Indigenous Peoples, and they are at once unique and connected. Each represents a sacred part of the whole. I'll share from my little part of the forest—the things I know, the things I'm coming to know, and some things that others have shared. Please take what you like and leave the rest.

What Is Wellness?

When I think of wellness, I think of health. The root of health is hāl, which means "to make whole." It is out of a harmonious whole that sacred qualities and gifts can begin to emerge to be shared with the community. Wellness, then, isn't just personal. What may begin as an individual pursuit becomes a noble way of being and living when it is developed to help the community.

Wellness, just like disease, affects everything around us. According to a Navajo Elder interviewed by Rupert Ross, all our actions are either hozhooji (moving toward harmony) or hashkeeji (moving toward disharmony). Notice that there is no third option, no suggestion that we can slide along in neutral, affecting nothing. Instead, the understanding is that whatever we do or say has an impact on everything around us, in one direction or another (Ross, 1996, p. 146).

Reflect and Respond
Write, draw, record, or explore these tasks:
- Identify three actions or behaviours that are moving you toward harmony or promoting your wellness.
- Identify three actions or behaviours that are moving you toward disharmony or discouraging your wellness.

Keep these actions and behaviours in mind as you explore wellness from the Indigenous perspective presented in this chapter.

Métis Elder Barbara Bruce remembers, when she was a child, people supporting each other in the community in a variety of ways, from physical labour, to planting medicine, to meeting basic needs. When I asked if there was a Michif word that conveyed this concept of supporting community well-being, she said it wasn't something that was discussed; it was just the way things were.

Métis writer Maria Campbell mirrors this notion: "Family [to our old people] meant sharing all things: wealth, knowledge, happiness and pain. It meant ... loving and caring enough about each other to be honest, and from that honesty, gathering strength to change those things which would hurt us all" (as cited in Macdougall, 2017, p. 9).

Elder Bruce offered the Cree/Michif word *wahkootowin*. Wahkootowin is a multifaceted concept that represents both our relationship with others and Creation and the way we should interact within those relationships. Thus, our path of wellness becomes a sacred responsibility, integrated with the path of the servant-leader. We honour this responsibility by becoming aware, and then taking action and making sacrifices so that we can work with and help others in a good way.

Wellness is about balance. I refer to the Sacred Hoop in understanding that my wellness is about finding balance in the Physical, Emotional, Mental, and Spiritual Directions. The Western world often looks at illness or wellness only from the physical aspect, whereas I try to keep myself grounded by practising a good life. I try to stay positive, eat right, exercise, and practise mindfulness and calmness. I do this by using my traditional way of living, as well as not swearing, smoking, or drinking. I go on the land as often as I can to harvest plants and animals and communicate with all of Creation. There, I give thanks for the things I have in life, as well as for the struggles and successes.

For me, the most important thing to be aware of is taking care of oneself. I must recognize when I am getting stressed and need to take time to rest and reenergize. I feel the need for this more when I do personal spiritual healing work, as I am drained afterwards, and get tossed and dragged by spirits when I try to sleep. This is when I know I have pushed myself to the edge.

I do not believe that society, in general, has a good grasp of wellness, because many people consider only the physical aspect. Mental health is still very stigmatized and misunderstood by all cultures.—*Elder Kipling*

Teachings on Wellness and the Sacred Circle

My first mentor was a woman who looked people in the eye and walked with dignity. At the time, I couldn't even look myself in the eye, and I walked with my head down and my hoodie up. She was a Sundancer who had learned about the culture in her later years. She knew about dreams and colours and living a clean life. I desperately wanted what she had. Once, she shared that the Sacred Circle took seven lifetimes to fully understand. So bear with me!

The Sacred Circle is shared in different ways among different Nations and teachers. I recall one Cree Knowledge Keeper sharing that as she grew up, the Sacred Circle wasn't spoken about—it was lived. In contrast, the Anishinaabe grandmother who taught me shared that her father would take her into their city yard and, using 36 pebbles, would make the Sacred Circle and share the teachings. I've learned that the Circle is a rich symbol of wholeness, change, and reconciliation.

We can use the Sacred Circle in our own way to explore the dimensions of our wellness.

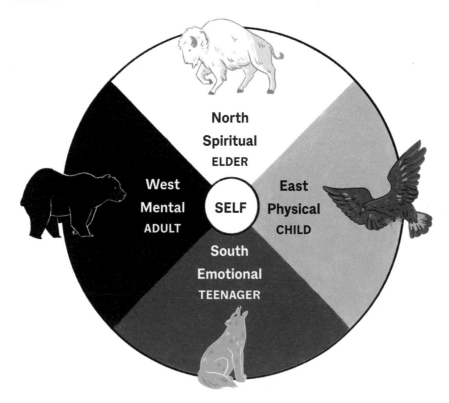

Recall the descriptions of the Four Directions: The *Physical dimension* is represented by the colour yellow, depicted by the rising sun and the gift of a brand-new day. Nourishing a healthy body through exercise, nutrition, and sleep are ways to promote physical wellness.

The *Emotional dimension* is represented by the colour red and represents the red-hot emotions we may sometimes have. Emotional wellness can come from being aware of, accepting, and expressing our feelings, and understanding the feelings of others.

The *Mental dimension* is represented by the colour black to depict our minds and the introspection it takes to journey through our lives. Engaging in the world through learning, problem-solving, and creativity can contribute to our mental wellness.

The *Spiritual dimension* is represented by the colour white, which symbolizes the harsh weather we must face and the wisdom of our Elders. The Spiritual is that which fills us up. It may mean connecting to our higher power, Creator, God, Buddha, Allah, or Nature, or whatever spirituality means to you.—*North Star*

Reflect and Respond
- Draw a circle with four quadrants. This will represent your Sacred Circle. Label each quadrant, starting in the East, with the Four Directions: Physical, Emotional, Mental, and Spiritual.
- Assess your level of well-being in each dimension. Colour in each quadrant to represent your assessment. A fully coloured quadrant represents fulfillment and health in that area. A partially coloured quadrant represents some work to be done.

In 2008, I was working at an insurance company. My life was a mess. I had connected with one of my clients, though, a middle-aged Ukrainian woman. Once, while visiting her office, I noticed a book on her shelf, *The Sacred Tree.* She told me I could have it. I didn't know about my Indigenous heritage at the time, but as I read, the words soaked into my bones. The Elders' words became like living, breathing teachers for me. I was thirsty for their messages of self-development, healing, and transformation.

At a time when I was in survival mode, disconnected from my potential, the following words awoke something in me: "Potentially, the seed has a mighty tree within it. The four aspects of our nature (Physical, Mental, Emotional, and Spiritual) are like seeds. They have the potential to grow into powerful Gifts" (Bopp et al., 1985, p. 13). These words helped me see that I didn't have to keep living the way I was living. That there were other possibilities. That I might have gifts underneath all the dross.

Respond and Reflect

The sacred task of imagining our ideal life gives us space to re-envision and rewrite our story of wellness. Let's catch a vision of your ideal life. Spend some time reflecting, writing, drawing, or collaging—any way you want to express what you see.

- What would it mean for you to be well physically? Which habits would you need to take up? Which habits would you need to release?
- What would it mean to be well emotionally? What practices could you include in your day to facilitate this? What would you need to let go of? (Explore relationships, work/home commitments, and so on.)
- What would it mean to be well mentally? What's your self-talk like? What can you put in place to support your vision?
- What would it mean to be well spiritually? What fills you up? What time-suckers would you need to release to create space for your story of wellness?

Wellness and Reconciliation

When I share my story, people often ask how I changed. As I dug into that question over the years, the answer that emerged is what I call my Integrated Reconciliation Framework. This model represents a process of holistic restoration. I think it's accessible for all but especially useful for those whose Circles have been broken by historical, social, familial, or internal dysfunction. The elements are:

- Relationships
- Reflection
- Readiness
- Reconstruction
- Restoration
- Reconciliation

The elements of this framework are interconnected like the elements of a tree in the forest, embedded within the Sacred Circle.

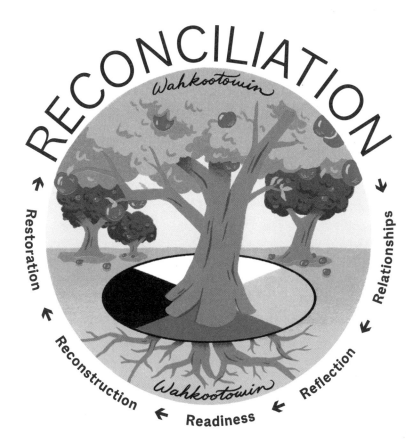

In this model, the tree represents us. Our *Relationships* with Creation, self, and other people are central to wellness. However, relationships also include our interconnection with cultural, social, economic, and social-emotional resources. In the image above, the soil, water, and sunshine represent relationships. Like soil, relationships hold us and nourish us. Water and sunshine feed our growth and sustain our process. This reflects wahkootowin, as described by Elder Bruce.

Thich Nhat Hanh, a Buddhist monk, noted that "when you plant lettuce, if it does not grow well, you don't blame the lettuce. You look for reasons it is not doing well. It may need fertilizer, or more water, or less sun" (Hanh, 1992, p. 78). In the same way, if the tree is not doing well, we must begin by examining the soil, the water, and the light sources. When we are unwell, we need to consider our relationships and resources to move along the path to wellness. For example, a tree planted in tight-packed soil won't do as well as a tree in loose soil. Similarly, if we are planted in tight relationships where we are not free to be who we truly are, or if the people in our relationships are toxic, our roots will not be able to get what they need. This affects the whole tree and the output of that tree. Likewise, without adequate light or water, a tree will starve. In the same way, if we do not have consistent access to cultural practices, basic needs, and strong communal social-emotional resources, we will decay.

Reflect and Respond
Make a T-chart. On one side, title Relationships, and on the other side, Resources.
- List your relationships that are harmonious and enjoyable—the ones that feed you.
- List resources that help you thrive. Remember that these include cultural, social, economic, and social-emotional resources, such as activities, connections, celebrations, and so on.

In this model, the roots of the tree are embedded into the Sacred Circle. Our relationships feed each aspect of our being. However, when we are embedded within relationship structures that are linked to historical trauma, other relational dysfunction, or poverty, our aspects of being struggle to grow and flourish. We become unbalanced and unwell, and we are unable to serve in a functional, sustainable way.

Through our relationships and resources, we begin to catch glimpses of what is possible. We can take time for *Reflection* on what we see. When I was 16 and living in a group home, I looked up to a worker there. She had a "risky" past, but came through, and was now helping high-risk girls. Although I wasn't aware of the process, being embedded in this positive relationship planted a seed—a vision that I could use my experiences to help others one day.

There came a time years later when I reached a place of *Readiness* to move toward that vision. *The Sacred Tree* states that:

> We gain a vision of what our potential is from our Elders and from the Teachings … [B]y trying to live up to that vision and by trying to live like the people we admire, we grow and develop. Our vision of what we can become is like a strong magnet pulling us toward it. (Bopp et al., 1985, p. 15)

Readiness is connected to initiative. We take courageous action, and our visions are propelled into reality, like seeds bursting into trees. Initiative helps us develop the parts of our Sacred Circle that are unbalanced.

I used to be a heavy smoker. Smoking affected every aspect of my life. It became clear that I needed to quit if I wanted to live long enough to be of service to others. After years of trying unsuccessfully, I eventually came to a place of readiness. I began again by searching for tips on how to quit cold turkey. I studied how the body rids itself of nicotine. I stuck inspirational quotes on sticky notes all over my apartment. I made a list of all the reasons I wanted to quit and envisioned what my life would be like as a non-smoker. My most important decision was to begin. It wasn't easy, but it felt like the right thing to do. I've now been smoke-free for years. I'm fit to serve.

Reflect and Respond

Choose something that you'd like to change—something that would make a big difference in your wellness in one of the four aspects, or Directions, of your nature. Focus on the questions below. You could write, draw, or attach images or quotes to each section.

- *Reflect:* Why and how is this element connected to your well-being? How does it affect each aspect of your Sacred Circle? When did you first notice you had an imbalance in this area? How does it affect your day-to-day life? How does it affect your ability and willingness to serve?
- *Vision:* What do you want this aspect of your life to look like, feel like, and be like? How might moving toward this vision affect the other aspects of your Circle? How might this new way of being affect your daily life? How might it affect your ability and willingness to serve others?
- *Readiness:* What will it take for you to be ready to act on this? What will your life be like next year if you choose not to move on it? What about in five years? Ten years? Forty years? What will your life be like if you choose to move on it?
- *Initiative:* What is a simple, concrete step that you're willing to take today to move toward your vision? What other steps will you need to take moving forward?

It is this process of reflection, vision, and readiness that fuels the process of *Reconstruction.* Like the growth of the tree trunk itself, outward and upward, reconstruction represents the health and balance of our Sacred Circle. At this stage, we release what is no longer working for us, and we adopt a new way of being. For years, I filled up on food and substances that were cheap, fast, and pleasurable. I walked around in constant fear and tension, feeling fundamentally unsafe, as if everything was an emergency. I couldn't regulate my emotions and impulses or maintain relationships or jobs. I was living in poverty (and I'm not just talking money here). My lifestyle created disharmony and affected everyone around me.

It has been a gradual process, but my lifestyle is fundamentally different today. It's harmonious and full. One by one, I released things that were causing suffering and craving and adopted new behaviours and habits. My mentor would encourage me to keep practising the new healthier ways of living. "They will become part of who you are," she'd say. Another mentor would remind me that "all behaviour is purposeful." My acting-out behaviours were meeting a Physical, Emotional, Mental, or Spiritual need. Then, my behaviours were unskillful—they led to disharmony, suffering, disconnection, and craving. Now, my behaviours are more skillful—they lead to harmony, peace, connection, and freedom.

I'll give another example. At the end of a busy workday, I'm exhausted. Sometimes, I deal with this by taking a 20-minute rest, playing with my paints, and having a call with a friend. This routine addresses my Physical, Emotional, Mental, and Spiritual needs, and I'm left peaceful. On other days, I've come home, lain on the couch with my phone to my face streaming videos, only getting up to prepare dinner and eat, and then it's back to the couch for more of the same. This routine seems to deal with my mental exhaustion, but it leaves me feeling restless, hungry, unproductive, and isolated.

Reflect and Respond

Let's make another T-chart. Label one side Unskillful and the other side Skillful.

- Make a list of some of your unskillful behaviours, the tricky ones that lead to issues—even though they seem to meet a need.
- Make a list of your skillful behaviours; they meet a need and you feel peaceful afterward. What do you notice?

Now, let's triage your lists:

- Choose the unskillful behaviour that's causing the most suffering and confusion in your life. What need is it meeting?
- Make a list of five other ways to meet that need.
- Put a star next to the one that you're willing to try this week. Write your choice(s) on sticky notes and place them around your home. On your cellphone, in the fridge, and on your steering wheel. Set alarms to remind you to practise the new behaviour.

Reconstruction takes place as we try on and embody health-promoting behaviours in each aspect or direction of our Circle. In the same way that night turns to light, change can be very subtle and gradual. Other times, it's abrupt, like a flash flood or thunderstorm.

My family has a history of heart disease, cancer, and diabetes. For me, sugar, flour, and processed foods are tricky and promote dis-ease. I decided to cut them out—hard and fast—replacing them with whole, earthy foods. In contrast, my spiritual practices have developed over time. I remember putting on a ribbon skirt and sitting quietly, soaking in the voice of the Elder during my first Pipe Ceremony. It brought something new into my Spiritual, Emotional, and Mental realms, and opened me up to a more disciplined practice of singing, dancing, praying, and meditating.

Sometimes, when we deal with the "kingpin" habit, that habit has other enforcing habits that naturally fall away. Some people will release an unskillful behaviour and find that their home is mysteriously tidier, they're exercising more, eating more nutritiously, and their family time is yummier. We begin to see wahkootowin in our daily habits. When I changed the way I ate, I became more stable emotionally, I had greater mental clarity, and my meditations became clearer and more consistent. All Four Directions were affected.

As we restore our Physical, Emotional, Mental, and Spiritual aspects, we begin to develop gifts related to the Four Directions. We are nourished by our relationships and resources: by Elders, Knowledge Keepers, guides, and mentors, by our community and the cultural and Ancestral teachings that surround us. The gifts mature and are renewed by our willingness to serve and work on ourselves. As I healed and cleaned up physically, I began to develop my ability to write, listen, and recognize connections in a big-picture way.

Reflect and Respond
- Throughout your week, take photographs of ways in which you take care of yourself physically, emotionally, mentally, and spiritually.
- Print your photos and make a Sacred Circle collage.

In time, this process of whole healing and restoration creates a baseline of wellness that prepares us to give back—to serve as a leader—sustainably. Wahkootowin represents this responsibility to live in a good way. Our gifts grow into fruit that, once ripened, are shared. This fruit drops back into the ground, enriching other relationships. Through our gifts, others in past, present, and future generations are blessed, nourished, and healed. New seeds are planted, and the community is fertilized.

This, I believe, is the gift of *Reconciliation*—a bringing together of past and future, of the bits and pieces of ourselves. This reconciliation happens first within a person. Then, as that integrated energy is absorbed and then shared, it affects the surrounding "forest": the family, the community, and, ultimately, the nation.

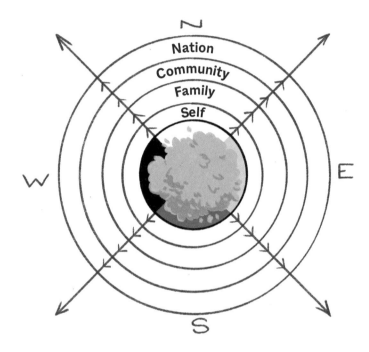

Through this series of processes, we travel around the Sacred Circle repeatedly. Healing is never-ending. We can revisit our vision, decide to change and grow, and choose to give back and lead again and again.

Wellness naturally emerges from a balanced way of being, in the same way that leaves and fruit emerge from a healthy tree. To be a servant-leader, there's an element of sacrifice. You sacrifice a quick pleasure for something that will lead to dynamic wellness later; you sacrifice and let go of time-worn habits for a greater good. As more of us have reconciled ourselves, more of us will be sharing the wholeness that naturally emerges from that state. As we share the fruit—that goodness—those seeds will be planted. Not just for us and our communities and families, but for coming generations.

Research now shows that although trauma causes disharmony and disruption to the brain, body, and DNA, choosing to live a health-promoting, harmonious lifestyle reverses such damage. This is not just for the individual but also for future generations (University of Zurich, 2016). My first spiritual mentor taught me that as I healed and walked this journey to wholeness, I was healing myself. But I was also healing my Ancestors—my father, grandfather, and grandmother whose Circles were broken, the people who couldn't restore and rebuild their own. She said I was restoring the Circle for them, the Old ones, but also for the future ones, the Young ones not yet here. What a blessing this is.

Closing Thoughts

This journey to wellness—to Integrated Reconciliation—is a messy, sacred responsibility. It's for all people, regardless of ethnicity, age, religion, lack of religion, gender, socioeconomic status, or job title. This is wahkootowin.

I'm walking this journey home. I'm coming home as a whole, healthy, proud Métis woman. I'm doing the work to move toward my highest and cleanest potential. I'm walking toward a peaceful, generous, harmonious way of living. This internal work will show up externally, healing, changing, and balancing all aspects of my life and relations. This is where I can give and share from, a full and fruitful Circle, as it was for my people way, way back. This is wahkootowin.

I believe that if enough of us do this work individually, our homes, our communities, and ultimately our nation will move toward Truth and Reconciliation. It's just a matter of time. I invite you, fellow traveller, to step into your Sacred Circle, respectfully, resiliently, and valiantly. See what's there. Muck around. Change what you can. Release what you can't. And then repeat. Restore your Circle.

References and Further Reading

TED. (2009, October 7). *The danger of a single story* | Chimamanda Adichie [Video, 19:16]. YouTube. https://www.youtube.com/watch?v=D9Ihs241zeg&vl=en

Bopp, J., Bopp, M., Brown, L., & Lane, P., Jr. (1985). *The sacred tree: Reflections on Native American spirituality*. Lotus Light Publications.

Dell, C. A., et al. (2015). *Connecting with culture: Growing our wellness* [Facilitators' handbook]. University of Saskatchewan, Research Chair in Substance Abuse.

Global Wellness Institute. (n.d.). *What is wellness?* Retrieved May 1, 2021, from https://globalwellnessinstitute.org/what-is-wellness/

Government of Western Australia. (2015). *WA health and wellbeing framework 2015–2030.* https://ww2.health.wa.gov.au/-/media/Files/Corporate/general-documents/Aboriginal-health/PDF/12853_WA_Aboriginal_Health_and_Wellbeing_Framework.pdf

Hanh, T. (1992). *Peace is every step: The path of mindfulness in everyday life.* Bantam Books.

Macdougall, B. (2017). *Land, family, and identity: Contextualizing Métis health and well-being.* National Collaborating Centre for Aboriginal Health. https://www.ccnsa-nccah.ca/docs/context/RPT-ContextualizingMetisHealth-Macdougall-EN.pdf

Millman, D. (1980). *The way of the peaceful warrior: A book that changes lives.* J Kramer.

Neufeld, L. (2022). We alchemists: Playing with pain, power, and potential [3-part article]. *Thriving Journal, 7*(5, 6, 7). https://growingedgetraining.com/thriving

———. (in press). *Cultivating the whole: An ecological exploration of creativity. Advancing creativity and innovation in education.* International Centre for Innovation in Education.

Ross, R. (1996). *Returning to the teachings: Exploring Aboriginal justice.* Penguin Books.

University of Zurich. (2016, June 23). Not only trauma but also the reversal of trauma is inherited. *ScienceDaily.* www.sciencedaily.com/releases/2016/06/160623120307.htm

Chapter 5

Physical Well-Being
Caring for Our Bodies with Compassion, Not by Comparison

Megan Hunter

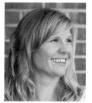

Megan Hunter, BKin, BEd, MSc (candidate), founder and social innovator at Peak + Prairie Co. Health Promotion, is on a mission to connect, create community, and collaborate with organizations, communities, and businesses to develop psychologically safe and healthy places where we play, live, and work. Megan credits her shift to psychological health promotion to her experience as a workplace wellness liaison with the Alberta School Employee Benefit Plan and many experiences shared with fellow education-sector employees. These days you can find Megan playing in the mountains on bikes and boards with her husband, Jon, and their newborn son.

> Comparison is the thief of joy.
> —*Theodore Roosevelt*

As an educator, I've been guilty of not drinking enough water in order to reduce bathroom breaks. I've skipped lunch to help students with math problems, forgone breakfast to arrive early at school for planning, and even missed dinner because I stayed too late helping a school club or team. I am sure some of this rings true for you, too. There have been times when I did not prioritize my physical health, and I paid the price for it. I became more susceptible to colds and had reduced energy from not sleeping enough, or from eating food that didn't make me feel my best. I also paid the price in reduced mobility, increased body pain, and a decline in my overall sense of well-being.

The times I felt the least at home in my skin were the stretches when I succumbed to diet culture and was over-exercising. I was surviving on copious amounts of coffee but very little nourishment. The sheer amount of activity took a toll on my body. I was constantly injured, yet still working out. I thought I was taking care of my body, yet, regardless of how I looked, I felt terrible. I did not have enough energy to be fully present or to redirect the mean thoughts I would regularly use to judge myself. For me, overworking and focusing on everyone else became an excuse for ignoring self-care. And my coping tool, for stress and life, was to over-exercise.

Whether you have overused your body, as I have, or underused it by being less physically active, you should notice when you are not respecting your body. Either way, both overuse and underuse are hurtful, not helpful. The journey to physical well-being is one of mindfulness to the body and "kindfulness" to ourselves.

The ironic thing is that, while I was over-exercising, I was working as a health educator, promoting physical health and activity. Yet I completely ignored my own professional knowledge and advice to others about the importance of rest and recovery.

Fast forward a few years to when I experienced a significant panic attack that took me off work for a month. It was after this initial collapse that I realized how crucial rest and recovery were to vitality. Over-scheduling myself, working to please others, and putting everyone else first, combined with too much physically taxing activity, was wearing me down, physically, mentally, and emotionally. There is no doubt that I was experiencing burnout. I had all the signs and symptoms and needed to find a way back to overall wellness.

Reflect and Respond
- Have there been times when you disregarded the needs of your body? What was your experience?
- What steps did you take, or are you taking, to overcome this challenge?

My necessary focus became caring for my whole self, including healthy physical care. I started with sleep, designing a routine that allowed me plenty of rest every night. The restful sleep helped lift the brain fog so that I could make better decisions about my wellness. I kept up my water intake to ensure hydration (also critical for good brain function) and began planning nutritious and satisfying meals.

 The Sacred Hoop is a good visual to remind us of the balance we need to maintain a healthy lifestyle. The Physical, Emotional, Mental, and Spiritual aspects of ourselves are constantly evolving throughout the day. Being aware of our needs is an important way to make sure we are getting what we need to teach and be happy. We know that when one aspect of the Sacred Hoop is out of balance, the others are as well, even if we are unaware of it.—*North Star*

I began to seek out health professionals who could help me manage the pain my body was in from overuse. I was careful to choose providers who had a holistic approach to health and were not focused on weight loss but instead emphasized caring for the total body. I'm thankful that my educator benefits allowed for top-notch care by trained professionals. I could get osteopathy to align my body's organs and structure, massage therapy for relaxation and muscle repair, physiotherapy for old injuries, acupuncture for hormone balance and sleep, and chiropractic for alignment.

One thing I learned from this process is that we do not have to live in pain. There are so many ways to address our concerns and prevent future injuries. The key was to give myself permission to reach out and get help. I needed to be the student this time and let myself be cared for.

Once I was rested, well-fed and hydrated, and free from pain, I was finally ready to incorporate intentional physical activity into my world. My goal was not to look a certain way but to feel good in my body, mind, and spirit. My movement now does not look as intense as it did. Activity has become about honouring my body. Some days it involves breathing exercises in bed. Other days, I'm lifting weights, stand-up paddle boarding, or attending a class at the gym, all for the joy of movement. I make decisions based on what makes sense for me that day and balance it with my mood, energy level, and responsibilities. Activity is now about experiencing the joy of movement. This has become essential to my well-being.

Along with the support I received for my physical well-being, I also worked with counsellors and therapists to attend to my mental health needs. They helped me to address issues such as self-worth and body image. This allowed me to find balance and harmony between the different elements of my life. As illustrated by the Sacred Hoop, I worked on becoming well Physically, Emotionally, Mentally, and Spiritually.

A New Paradigm for Physical Health

Many of us bust out the comparisons when it comes to rating our physical health. As a health educator for school employees, I've heard many stories from teachers over the years about how the demands of the job make being active and eating well exceptionally challenging during the school year. These professionals, even while acknowledging that their work can be highly emotional and mentally taxing, can be hard on themselves for forgetting to eat because they were so busy or not wanting to exercise after a long day. More concerning was the judgment I'd hear from teachers comparing themselves to others: "Mrs. K seems to have it all together! Her lunches are healthy, and she runs every day. But I am exhausted and feel like I am failing because I can't do it all and I don't fit into last year's jeans!"

Well, you don't need to fit into skinny jeans to be healthy. I have found it personally helpful to think of my own overall health in terms of my health habits, not my body shape or size. I feel better physically and mentally when I focus on being healthy instead of focusing on the numbers on a scale. Rather than comparing how much we weigh today with how much our neighbour weighs or how much we weighed last year, let's put the comparisons away and focus on a new way of thinking about our physical health.

The concept of self-compassion is introduced in chapter 2, "Permission to Be Well." I have learned along my journey that taking care of my body can be a powerful way to practise self-compassion. Too often, we treat the body using forms of punishment, thinking that they are beneficial. Restrictive diets, over-exercising, and not sleeping enough are some of the ways we try to fulfill our quest for perfection, comparing ourselves with some impossible ideal. However, these behaviours can affect our mood and relationships, and can also lead to binge eating, injuries, and burnout. What our bodies truly need are the compassion and care that we would recommend to anyone else. Our bodies do so much for us, and yet we spend so much time criticizing them. Our bumps, lumps, scars, wrinkles, and dimples are important parts of ourselves that tell our unique stories. They are gifts. We need to flip the paradigm from comparing our bodies to celebrating our bodies.

We know that physical health is about more than diet and body shape. It's about the experience of living in our bodies and how we feel, think, move, rest, repair, and fuel them. Amid the hustle and bustle of a school day, week, month, season, and year, how can you make your physical health a priority so that you have the energy and strength to be well?

Applying an 80-20 Mindset

When we apply 80-20 thinking to physical health, we are looking to follow healthy habits 80 percent of the time, and then allow ourselves 20 percent flexibility to relax. This 80-20 balance is especially effective in relation to nourishment and movement, and health experts attest to this mindset as a way to maintain physical health (Cutter, 2012). In addition, research suggests that people can maintain overall health by eating healthy most of the time, while enjoying some splurges (Ackermann et al., 2014). This study adds that you may also have a lower risk for conditions such as heart disease, high blood pressure, and cancer by following a balanced approach to health.

This mindset contrasts with all-or-nothing thinking. That kind of perfectionism leads us to think that we must adhere to rules 100 percent of the time. Everyone's health situation is different, and there are some habits that some of us really do need to stick to 100 percent of the time—like avoiding something we're allergic to! If in doubt, check with a health-care professional. But often, you may find that "most of the time" works. The benefit of treating ourselves well most of the time is that this provides a buffer that might be needed when you feel the pinch of time. For example, you may need that buffer when writing report cards, during a tough day at work, during a parent-teacher interview, or on the day when you have a full schedule. The 20 percent can also be for days when you don't want a schedule, or when you have to do something that may cause a deficit in your sleeping, eating, or movement patterns. With the 80-20 mindset, we challenge all-or-nothing approaches and practise self-compassion by being a little easier on ourselves.

Reflect and Respond
- In what ways have you experienced all-or-nothing thinking related to eating or physical movement?
- How does this impact sustaining healthy behaviours for you?
- How might an 80-20 mindset serve you?

Many Indigenous communities have ongoing intergenerational trauma to deal with in our daily lives. Residential schools and the Sixties Scoop have had negative consequences for Indigenous Peoples and their families. The pain that resulted from these institutions and policies has lingered on in our communities and in our bodies. I call this body memory, or blood memory. Even if a generation of children from a family didn't attend residential schools, the results are often the same in our bodies. This body memory reveals itself in the dis-eases we carry. (When we encounter disease in the body, it's our body in dis-ease. Our Sacred Circle is out of balance.) If the communities we live in are subjected to logging, water waste, and other harms, the results are the same. Our communities suffer from high diabetes rates, cancer, skin ailments, and many other conditions because of the government defiling the lands that we live on in our territories.

We are inheritors of these painful legacies, and so the results show up in our Physical, Emotional, Mental, and Spiritual bodies. Sometimes the stresses of everyday life weigh us down, and exercise and healthy eating are not something we can actively work toward every day. Many Indigenous Peoples practise Traditional Healing and attend ceremonies to help deal with the trauma inflicted upon us as a People.—*North Star*

Sleep and Well-Being

In May 2021, I became a mom for the first time at the age of 37. Before this new adventure, I had, for the most part, 37 years to sleep when I wanted for as long as I needed. As tough as it is now to get the sleep I need, I have to rest when I can, and also teach our son how to be a sleeper.

Why? Because sleep is foundational to our overall well-being. It is the time when our bodies reset us for the next day. Research shows that sleep is essential to overall mental health because it helps to improve memory, overall brain function, emotional regulation, hormone regulation, stress response, and resilience (Harvard Health, 2021).

Practising the habits of sleep hygiene is one way to ensure that we are taking restful care of ourselves. It is critical to our overall wellness to develop a sleep routine, especially a good bedtime routine.

If you have difficulty sleeping or have never prioritized sleep, here are some helpful guidelines (Suni, 2022):

- Choose a realistic amount of time that you want to sleep each night (seven, eight, or nine hours).
- Consider when you have to wake up in the morning. Determine your bedtime accordingly.
- Plan for 30 minutes of device- and screen-free time before bed. Blue light from screens reduces melatonin, a chemical that your brain needs for sleep.
- Plan an unwinding activity such as reading, stretching or other light movements, teatime, or a warm bath. (Avoid intense exercise just before bedtime.)
- When possible, allow at least two hours from your last meal to bedtime to aid digestion, reduce heartburn, and avoid feeling too full to sleep.
- Try to maintain a regular sleep schedule. Once you have determined your bed- and wake times, try to stay within 30 minutes of these times each morning and night.
- As much as you are able, keep your bedroom dark and cool for optimal sleep.
- If you wake in the night, to avoid activating your mind, try not to look at the time.
- If you are using your phone as your alarm and it increases the likelihood of checking messages right before bed, in the night, or before you crawl out of bed, switch your phone for an alarm clock.

Children and Our Sleep

Our sleep patterns are, of course, influenced by those with whom we live. If we are caregivers, it is often challenging to get enough sleep, whether we are caring for a baby, toddler, child, or teen. We need to consider how to ensure our children get enough sleep, but also attend to our own sleep needs.

Good sleep hygiene is advised for children. The Canadian Pediatric Society (<https://cps.ca/>) recommends 12 to 16 hours of sleep for infants, 11 to 14 hours for toddlers, 10 to 13 hours for ages three to five, 9 to 12 hours for ages six to twelve, and 8 to 10 hours for teenagers. Consistency is important, as are preparing the space and establishing pre-sleep routines such as non-screen time, brushing teeth, washing, and bedtime stories (Canadian Pediatric Society, 2017).

Of course, when children have challenges sleeping, that causes challenges for you as well. Whether a child is ill and keeps you up at night, or whether sleep patterns are the issue, your self-care can help you cope. As much as possible, try to sleep while your child sleeps, share nighttime duties when possible, and be gentle with yourself with other responsibilities. (Maybe you can give yourself permission to hold off on a few household chores in order to rest.)

Establishing effective routines for sleep hygiene is an important part of promoting our positive mental health and well-being. No matter what age, we all need sleep, both to be at our best and to allow our bodies time to recover and keep us well.

Reflect and Respond

Think about your habits, activities, and goals for good rest.

- What time do you ideally wish to start your bedtime routine?
- What responsibilities do you have before your bedtime routine? (For example, kids, lunches, tidying.)
- How do you begin your bedtime routine? What activities prepare you for bed? (For example, put out clothing for the next day.)
- To promote optimal sleep, which of the following will you do? (Check all that apply.)
  - ☐ Spend at least 30 minutes away from screens and devices.
  - ☐ Start my bedtime routine early enough to be in bed at my preferred time.
  - ☐ Pause when I have the impulse to do tasks that can wait until the next day.
  - ☐ Make the room dark and cool.
  - ☐ Have required accessories to help me sleep (for example, earplugs, eye mask, nose strips).
  - ☐ Write down any thoughts or to-do items for the next day so that I do not dwell on them.
  - ☐ Set an alarm to the appropriate wake-up time for an average of 8 hours of sleep.
  - ☐ Plan to do a calming activity, such as meditation or breathing, to relax my mind.
  - ☐ Other

Nourishment

Like sleep, nourishment is key to our well-being. Research indicates that "good nutrition is associated with better mental health outcomes, whereas a poor diet is associated with a greater risk of depression and anxiety" (Be You, 2021).

Unfortunately, media often gives us confusing messages about the perfect way to eat. These messages can lead to getting caught up in the latest dieting crazes. The problem is that many of these approaches are not sustainable and do not promote a positive relationship with food. If you find it difficult to sift through the messages, consider talking to a dietitian or nutritionist who can help you learn about positive and sustainable approaches to nourishment.

So, what is good nutrition? The food we eat is fuel for the activities we do. It is nourishment for function and pleasure. However, foods are often labelled as being good or bad, and this makes it difficult to make healthy and enjoyable choices. Instead of labelling food, try noticing what you put in your body and how you feel after you eat it. This is an example of practising mindfulness through everyday life. Notice how you feel when you prepare, buy, and try certain foods. Take note of foods you enjoy eating and foods that make you feel fuelled and nourished. Consider choosing one meal each day at which you want to be extra mindful. For example, at breakfast, focus on each sip of your morning beverage and notice the sleepy start of the morning or the hustle and bustle in your household. There is no need to judge it; just notice and enjoy the moment. This everyday mindfulness can transform our relationship with food. It can help us to know what we like and dislike, when we are still hungry, and when we are satisfied.

Intuitive eating is similar in many ways to mindful eating. This approach to health and food "has nothing to do with diets, meal plans, discipline, or willpower," as Alana Kessler explains it. Instead, it focuses on "how to get in touch with your body cues," such as "hunger, fullness, and satisfaction, while learning to trust your body around food" (Kessler, 2019).

Make Mindful Food Choices

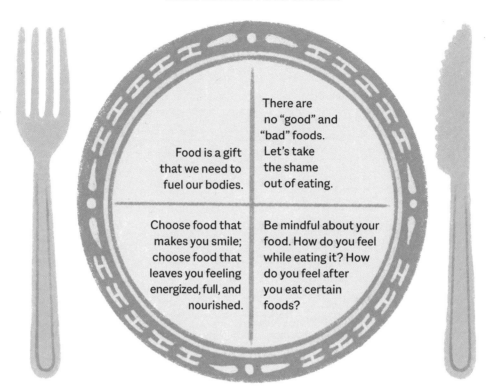

Food is a gift that we need to fuel our bodies.

There are no "good" and "bad" foods. Let's take the shame out of eating.

Choose food that makes you smile; choose food that leaves you feeling energized, full, and nourished.

Be mindful about your food. How do you feel while eating it? How do you feel after you eat certain foods?

 Our Indigenous communities are often removed from city centres, and the fresh produce is either hard to come by or extremely expensive. When we are living with poverty, we are immersed in dysfunction and will often try to subdue our pain by overindulging in different things. This may eventually lead to dis-ease. Without proper access to fresh produce and other healthy food choices in our communities, we switch out fresh, healthy foods for processed foods that are easier to get hold of and are less expensive. Also, when living with stress, we may choose processed foods because they are quicker to make.

There are programs in some of our communities that support gardening and nutrition for those living with dis-ease. Land-based education for Indigenous families is important for sustaining a healthy diet that comes from the land

and supports body health. This leads to a traditional diet, which is healthier and promotes physical activity as well as food sovereignty.

Indigenous Peoples regularly hold community feasts that take place during births, deaths, and other important ceremonies throughout the year. For the Sundance, for example, communities gather before and after to share time together and celebrate the Sundancers giving of themselves for healing. Traditional foods such as fish, wild rice, corn, wild meat, and berries are an important element of these celebrations. These foods are sacred to us as Indigenous Peoples and are harvested in a respectful way.—*North Star*

Planning for Nourishment

Another way we can set ourselves up for positive eating experiences is by thinking about and planning what we will eat each week. You may find these planning tools helpful. Remember the 80-20 guideline. Your plan doesn't have to be perfect, and you don't need to follow the plan impeccably.

Reflect and Respond

This activity can be used for weekly nutrition planning. You can use it to be reflective and prepare for the week ahead, while still having flexibility.

- What is your nutrition focus for the week?
  - ☐ To pause daily to eat lunch.
  - ☐ To eat seasonal fruits and vegetables.
  - ☐ To choose a variety of foods that make me feel good.
  - ☐ To fuel my body for energy to get me through the week.
  - ☐ Other
- What is going on this week? Are there days when someone else is preparing meals or when you plan to eat out?
- Is there something you can prepare in bulk over the weekend to save time?
- Who can help or support you in planning and preparing this week? Do you have to do this all on your own or can you enlist your family?

- How will you get the items you need? Can you order groceries online or plan with a friend to meet at a farmers' market?
- What activities are you doing each day, and will these foods provide enough energy?

Consider sketching out a weekly meal plan to stay on track with your nutrition goals. The aim is not to give you another thing to do, but rather to save the stress of rushing home hungry, not knowing what to cook, and feeling pressured to find something nutritious to feed yourself (and possibly others while being asked, "What's for dinner?").

Follow up on your meal plan with a detailed grocery list.

You may want to investigate various useful applications for your phone, tablet, or laptop that can help support your nutrition goals. Many not only help you with meal planning, but they also suggest recipes and generate grocery lists. Some apps that I have found useful (at the time of first printing) are Paprika, Mealtime, and MealPrepPro. If you are interested in mindful eating, there are apps for that as well (Am I Hungry?, Eat Drink and Be Mindful, and Mindful Eating Tracker). Similarly, there are apps focusing on intuitive eating (Peace with Food, Insight Timer, and Cara). For further information on nutrition, check out Canada's Food Guide (<https://food-guide.canada.ca/en/>).

There are many approaches and resources available to support nourishing our bodies. Choose what feels right to you, in consultation with your doctor. Consider focusing on taking care of your body and respecting it for all that it has to offer you.

Disordered Eating

A disordered relationship with food can compromise your overall physical and mental health. Since the pandemic, eating disorders have risen in children, adolescents, and adults (Zipfel et al., 2022). Here are some Canadian-based resources if you or a loved one need support. Please reach out for help.

- Canadian Eating Disorder Alliance (<https://edfc.ca/resources-2/>)
- Canadian Mental Health Association (<https://cmha.ca/mental-health/understanding-mental-illness/eating-disorders>)
- National Eating Disorder Information Centre (<https://nedic.ca/>)

Hydration

Drinking enough water each day is important to our overall wellness. Water helps to regulate body temperature, keep joints lubricated, prevent infections, deliver nutrients to cells, and keep organs functioning properly. Being well-hydrated also improves sleep quality, cognition, and mood. Research has shown the significant role that hydration plays in positive mental health, including feeling calmer, less depressed, and more mindfully alert (Masento et al., 2014).

Teachers tend to live by timetables and from task to task. We rush to and from class in response to the bells and must wait for the bell to take a washroom break. We stop to talk to a student who needs help and try to cram in prep time and marking between periods. This busyness may lead us to forget about or limit water intake. At times, I have been guilty of this myself. I need to be mindful of hydration to function at my best. Try to make a good-sized water bottle your friend and aim to drink eight to ten cups (two to two and a half litres) throughout the day, plus an extra half-litre for every hour of exercise you do.

 Indigenous People have a healthy relationship with water. This was our main daily drink and was also used to make teas, not only to sip and enjoy but also as medicine. Water was the basis for all our cooking and healing medicines. To this day, the Anishinaabe honour water daily, as well as in our ceremonies. One particular ceremony is called the Sweat Lodge Ceremony. We heat up rocks in the sacred fire and put them inside the Sweat Lodge, which is covered up with tarps. Water, which we refer to as medicine, is poured on the heated rocks to help us sweat out impurities in our bodies.

Many Indigenous communities do not have access to clean water, and First Nations communities across Canada still have long-term drinking water advisories (Government of Canada, 2022). The city of Winnipeg receives its drinking water from Shoal Lake, and yet the Shoal Lake First Nation could not access clean drinking water from the lake and was under a water advisory for more than 20 years.

Water is life and a way of life for many Indigenous Peoples, yet corporations pollute the waters surrounding their communities. Clear-cutting of forests and dumping wastewater and human waste pollutes waters to the point of killing lakes, rivers, and other tributaries. Our ceremonial teachings tell us that water is sacred, yet many First Nations communities still struggle with this basic need.—*North Star*

Managing Pain

Pain affects not only our ability to exercise and participate in activities of daily living but also our overall mood and wellness. Pain is often associated with mental health conditions such as anxiety and depression. "Living with daily pain is physically and emotionally stressful. Chronic stress is known to change the levels of stress hormones and neurochemicals found within your brain and nervous system; these can affect your mood, thinking and behavior" (Mental Health America, n.d.). Rest and recovery are essential to managing pain and important to our physical health and overall wellness.

Reflect and Respond
- How does pain make you feel?
- Finish the sentence: When I am in pain, I _____.
- Ask your pain what it needs. (For example, rest, a massage, physiotherapy.)
- Identify resources you have to help you deal with pain. (For example, employee benefit plans, private health plans, public health professionals.)
- Prioritize healing. Rest and follow the advice of your health professional team.
- You may require certain exercises to strengthen and retrain your body. Take the time for this and think of it as an investment in your future.

Mindful Movement

Active movement is something we all do every day. A teacher may take thousands of steps from class to class, climb stairs, and participate in movement activities with their students, and yet they often beat themselves up for not exercising. We must change that mindset to see movement as an active, joyful choice that benefits our overall well-being.

Research has demonstrated the effectiveness of physical movement in managing mental health. "Physical activity stimulates brain chemicals that leave you feeling happier, more relaxed and less anxious" (Mayo Clinic, 2021). Movement also makes us feel more energetic and helps us to sleep better. Remember the Sacred Hoop:

physical activity affects holistic well-being by supporting us, not only Physically, but also Emotionally, Mentally, and Spiritually.

As with nutrition, there's very little good or bad when it comes to how we move our bodies. The activity that is best for you is the one that you'll do and enjoy, and the one that feels good in your body.

Are you starting to notice a pattern? It is ultimately most important that you feel good in your body. Yes, pain sometimes prevents us from moving the way we want to. But when our pain is managed, when we are well-hydrated, nourished, and rested, we get the most out of our movement. Activity can also help us feel our best by lifting our spirits, getting us outdoors in the sunshine and fresh air, and oftentimes interacting with others.

 Many Indigenous Peoples participate in something that I call sacred movement. The Anishinaabe have many healing ceremonies that were derived from our teachings given to us by our animal teachers. I think especially of the many Bird Dances in spring and the Figure Eight Dance of the bee. These dances were the basis of our sacred ceremonial dances. When Sundancing, we dance from sun-up to sundown, fasting for four days. We have healing dances such as the jingle dress dance you see at a Pow Wow, and we dance for healing in other ceremonies. Again, all these ceremonies take place outside, helping us connect to each other and the land.—*North Star*

Reflect and Respond

Take a moment to identify the movement that fits into your life and feels good!

- What do you enjoy? List physical activities you look forward to doing and that make you happy even if you haven't been able to do them lately. Does a nature walk help you feel more connected to yourself? Does a swim have you glowing afterward?
- What feels good for your body? Try to avoid listing movement you only think you should do. For example, if you used to be a runner but it hasn't felt great in some time, give yourself permission to choose a different activity.

- What do you have access to? Think about walking or rolling paths, music, other people, online subscriptions, and free programs online or in the community.
- Who do you want to enjoy these activities with? Is there a friend you love to walk and talk with or an existing community you can join?
- How do the seasons affect how you move? A benefit of being in Canada is the changes in seasons and weather. Having activities we do in certain weather can be motivational and helps us look forward to a season we may have otherwise dreaded.
- How do you plan to recover? Recovery makes us better at movement and at repairing and replenishing our muscles and energy stores. And yes, a monthly massage can be part of your movement plan.

As important as movement is, we must still put our well-being first, practise self-compassion, and give ourselves permission to do only what is best for us. Always consider your present condition when deciding whether to exercise. Use the exercise decision tool, How Do I Move Today? (on the following page) to help you make that choice.

Workplace Wellness and Physical Well-Being

Throughout this book, you will find many suggestions for strategies for self-care that you, as an educator, can consider adopting individually. But we recognize that there must also be systems-level responsibility for educator well-being. Employers are obligated to create workplaces that foster the psychological and physical well-being of employees.

Research suggests that initiatives taken by employers to address the physical well-being of staff have a significant valuable effect on their mental health. Organizations that promoted physical activity in the workplace saw higher levels of concentration, reduced stress, and improved creativity among staff (Hogan et al., 2013). Whether this activity was scheduled yoga classes, organized walks, or team sports, staff reported both physical and mental improvements.

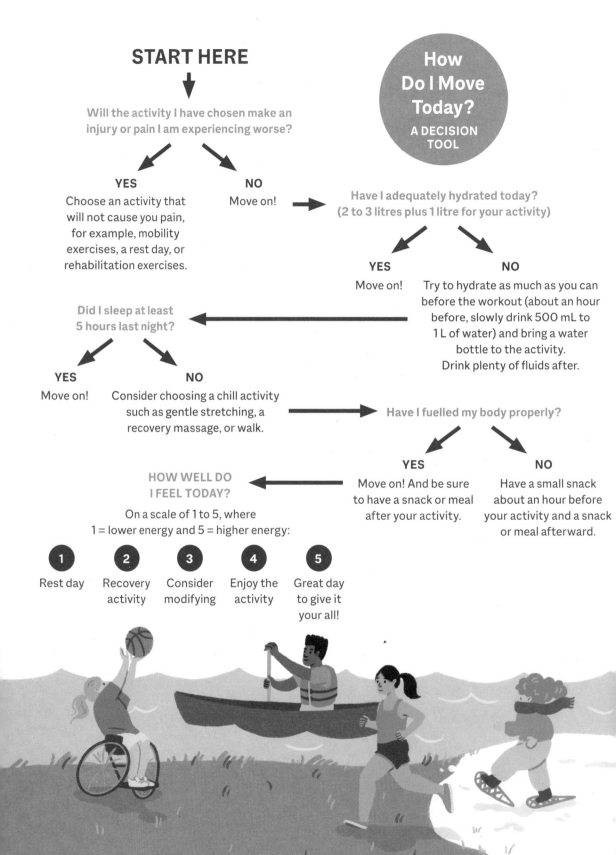

START HERE

How Do I Move Today?
A DECISION TOOL

Will the activity I have chosen make an injury or pain I am experiencing worse?

YES
Choose an activity that will not cause you pain, for example, mobility exercises, a rest day, or rehabilitation exercises.

NO
Move on!

Have I adequately hydrated today? (2 to 3 litres plus 1 litre for your activity)

YES
Move on!

NO
Try to hydrate as much as you can before the workout (about an hour before, slowly drink 500 mL to 1 L of water) and bring a water bottle to the activity. Drink plenty of fluids after.

Did I sleep at least 5 hours last night?

YES
Move on!

NO
Consider choosing a chill activity such as gentle stretching, a recovery massage, or walk.

Have I fuelled my body properly?

YES
Move on! And be sure to have a snack or meal after your activity.

NO
Have a small snack about an hour before your activity and a snack or meal afterward.

HOW WELL DO I FEEL TODAY?

On a scale of 1 to 5, where 1 = lower energy and 5 = higher energy:

1 Rest day
2 Recovery activity
3 Consider modifying
4 Enjoy the activity
5 Great day to give it your all!

In the same way, workplaces that promote healthy nutrition see the benefits, not just for physical health, but also for workplace well-being. Studies have found that the workplace environment can positively influence the health of its employees by, for example, providing adequate time for staff to eat at a relaxed pace and by offering healthy food choices and snacks at staff meetings and professional development workshops (Meridian Wellness, 2018).

Leaders at the school and division or district level have the power to boost the well-being of staff. For more about fostering workplace wellness and psychological health and safety in the workplace, see chapter 13, "An Invitation for Leaders in Education: Creating Psychologically Safe Work Environments."

Closing Thoughts

One thing I have learned from spending hours in one-on-one health sessions with educators is that we all struggle to properly care for ourselves. There is no perfect routine. When you let go of unrealistic expectations, you can begin to make decisions for your body and what it needs. We get only one body to take us through life—treat it with the care and kindness you deserve.

Reflect and Respond

Think about your physical well-being from a holistic perspective.

- What actions can you initiate today to promote your own wellness in relation to:
  - Sleep _____
  - Nourishment _____
  - Hydration _____
  - Managing pain _____
  - Movement _____
- Close your eyes, take three deep breaths, and let your body relax.
- Envision yourself taking these actions with self-compassion and mindfulness.

References and Further Reading

Academy of Nutrition and Dietetics, Dietitians of Canada, and the American College of Sports Medicine. (2016). Nutrition and athletic performance [Joint position statement]. *Medicine & Science in Sports & Exercise, 48*(3), 543–68. https://journals.lww.com/acsm-msse/Fulltext/2016/03000/Nutrition_and_Athletic_Performance.25.aspx

Ackermann, G., Kirschner, M., Guggenbühl, L., Abel, B., Klohn, A., & Mattig, T. (2015). Measuring success in obesity prevention. *Obesity Facts, 8*(1), 17–29. https://doi.org/10.1159/000374082

Be You. (2021). *Nutrition and mental health.* https://beyou.edu.au/fact-sheets/wellbeing/nutrition-and-mental-health

Bergland, C. (2017, July 18). Silent third-person talk facilitates emotion regulation. *Psychology Today.* https://www.psychologytoday.com/ca/blog/the-athletes-way/201707/silent-third-person-self-talk-facilitates-emotion-regulation

Canadian Mental Health Association. (n.d.). *Eating disorders* [Brochure]. https://cmha.ca/mental-health/understanding-mental-illness/eating-disorders

Canadian Pediatric Society. (2017, December). *Healthy sleep for your baby and child.* Caring for kids. https://caringforkids.cps.ca/handouts/healthy-living/healthy_sleep_for_your_baby_and_child

Couturier J., Pellegrini, D., Miller, C., Bhatnagar, N., Boachie, A., Bourret, K., Brouwers, M., Coelho, J. S., Dimitropoulos, G., Findlay, S., Ford, C., Geller, J., Grewal, S., Gusella, J., Isserlin, L., Jericho, M., Johnson, N., Katzman, D. K., Kimber, M., … Webb, C. (2020). *The COVID-19 pandemic and eating disorders in children, adolescents, and emerging adults: Recommendations from the Canadian Consensus Panel.* Canadian Institute of Health Research. https://cihr-irsc.gc.ca/e/52053.html

Cutter, T. (2012). *The 80/20 diet* (2nd ed.). Healthy Chef.

Eating Disorders Foundation of Canada. (n.d.). *Resources: Canadian Eating Disorder Alliance (CEDA).* Retrieved September 12, 2021, from https://edfc.ca/resources-2/

Fortier, M., McFadden, T., & Faulkner, G. (2020). Evidence-based recommendations to assist adults with depression to become lifelong movers. *Health Promotion and Chronic Disease Prevention in Canada, 40*(10), 299–308. https://doi.org/10.24095/hpcdp.40.10.01

Gene. (2021, March 14). Serious question: Should you exercise while sick? *GymStreak Blog.* https://blog.gymstreak.com/should-you-exercise-while-sick/

Government of Canada. (2022). *Remaining long-term drinking water advisories.* https://www.sac-isc.gc.ca/eng/1614387410146/1614387435325

Harvard Health. (2021). Sleep and mental health: Sleep deprivation can affect your mental health. *Harvard Health Blog*. https://www.health.harvard.edu/newsletter_article/sleep-and-mental-health

Hogan, C. L., Mata, J., & Carstensen, L. L. (2013). Exercise holds immediate benefits for affect and cognition in younger and older adults. *Psychology and Aging*, *28*(2), 587–94. https://doi.org/10.1037/a0032634

Kessler, A. (2019). *Intuitive eating 101*. Be Well. https://www.bewellbyak.com/writings/Intuitive-eating

Masento, N., Golightly, M., Field, D., Butler, L., & van Reekum, C. (2014). Effects of hydration status on cognitive performance and mood. *British Journal of Nutrition*, *111*(10), 1841–52. https://doi.org/10.1017/S0007114513004455

Mayo Clinic. (2021). *Exercise: 7 benefits of regular physical activity*. Mayo Foundation for Medical Education and Research. https://www.mayoclinic.org/healthy-lifestyle/fitness/in-depth/exercise/art-20048389

Mental Health America. (n.d.). *Chronic pain and mental health*. Retrieved September 1, 2021, from https://www.mhanational.org/chronic-pain-and-mental-health

Meridian Wellness. (2018, September 12). Eating well at work. *Better Mental Health Magazine*. https://bmhmag.com/eating-well-at-work/

Michaelides, A., & Zis, P. (2019). Depression, anxiety and acute pain: Links and management challenges. *Postgrad Med*, *131*(7), 438–44. https://doi.org/10.1080/00325481.2019.1663705

Moser, J. S., Dougherty, A., Mattson, W. I., Katz, B., Moran, T. P., Guevarra, D., Shablack, H., Ayduk, O., Jonides, J., Berman, M. G., & Kross, E. (2017). Third-person self-talk facilitates emotion regulation without engaging cognitive control: Converging evidence from ERP and fMRI. *Scientific Reports*, *7*(4519). https://doi.org/10.1038/s41598-017-04047-3

Ortiz, R., Elder, A., Elder, C., & Dawes, J. (2019). A systematic review on the effectiveness of active recovery interventions on athletic performance of professional-, collegiate-, and competitive-level adult athletes. *Journal of Strength and Conditioning Research*, *33*(8), 2275–87. https://doi.org/10.1519/JSC.0000000000002589

Penney, T. L., & Kirk, S. F. (2015). The health at every size paradigm and obesity: Missing empirical evidence may help push the reframing obesity debate forward. *American Journal of Public Health*, *105*(5), e38–e42. https://doi.org/10.2105/AJPH.2015.302552

Quinn, E. (2021, November 8). *Why you need rest and recovery after exercise*. Verywell fit. https://www.verywellfit.com/the-benefits-of-rest-and-recovery-after-exercise-3120575

Suni, E. (2022, March 11). *Healthy sleep tips*. Sleep Foundation. https://www.sleepfoundation.org/sleep-hygiene/healthy-sleep-tips

Swartzendruber, K. (2013, October 8). *The importance of rest and recovery for athletes*. Michigan State University Extension. https://www.canr.msu.edu/news/the_importance_of_rest_and_recovery_for_athletes

Taylor, K., & Jones, E. B. (2022, May). *Adult dehydration*. StatPearls. https://www.ncbi.nlm.nih.gov/books/NBK555956/

University Health Network. (2022). *Helpful hints for better sleep* [Brochure]. https://www.uhn.ca/PatientsFamilies/Health_Information/Health_Topics/Documents/Helpful_Hints_for_Better_Sleep.pdf

Vitale, K. C., Owens, R., Hopkins, S. R., & Malhotra, A. (2019). Sleep hygiene for optimizing recovery in athletes: Review and recommendations. *International Journal of Sports Medicine*, *40*(8), 535–43. https://doi.org/10.1055/a-0905-3103

Zipfel, S., Schmidt, U., & Giel, K. E. (2022, January). The hidden burden of eating disorders during the COVID-19 pandemic. *Lancet Psychiatry*, 9, 9–11. https://doi.org/10.1016/S2215-0366(21)00435-1

Chapter 6

Just Breathe
Strategies for Well-Being
Cher Brasok

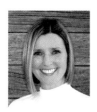 **Cher Brasok** is the founder of Connect to your Calm. When stress destroyed her health, Cher's recovery depended on her learning how to better cope. Her path back to health included studying and putting into practice what she learned from experts in positive psychology, Western medicine, Eastern medicine, naturopathic medicine, and mindfulness. Now that she is a successful entrepreneur, stress still happens, but she deals with it differently. Cher is on a mission to share what she knows about wellness and coping with stress, all to help people develop healthy habits for their physical and emotional well-being.

> When you own your breath,
> nobody can steal your peace.
> —*Anonymous*

Stress is an interesting thing. Ten years ago, if someone had asked me to describe my life, stressful is not a word I would have used. Busy, yes. I was so tuned out and caught up in the busyness of my life that I wasn't paying attention to how I was feeling. Then boom! I got sick, really sick, and stress was the culprit. Stress had destroyed my physical and mental health.

My path back to wellness included exploring, learning, and using a variety of tools to help me better cope when feeling overwhelmed, anxious, or stressed out. This led to opportunities to share my newly learned skills with family, friends, and, eventually, with students, teachers, and school staff. It has been a journey indeed.

It all started with the sentence: "I don't know what else I can do for you." This one sentence changed my life in a way I could never have imagined. After six months of running every medical test he could think of and sending me to specialists, my family doctor had nothing else to suggest. I was thankful that he found no sign of disease anywhere, yet my physical and mental health were at an all-time low.

Now what? With a beautiful young family at home and so much life ahead of me, I refused to stop looking for answers. One of my dearest friends reached out and asked if I had ever considered seeing a naturopathic doctor. I had never heard of a naturopath before, but I was open to anything at that point. Within a matter of days, I had an appointment and was on the beginning of a new path to wellness.

I arrived for my first appointment having no idea what to expect. I soon learned that naturopaths practise an alternative approach to health that differs from medical science. Dr Bunzenmeyer welcomed me into her office, and I instantly felt at ease. "So, what brings you here today?" she asked. I burst into tears and told her the whole story of how I was feeling and what had been going on. She asked questions about my life, lifestyle, stressors, and medical history. I was blown away by the thoroughness of her questioning, her gentle presence, and her empathic listening.

She then introduced me to two terms I had never heard before: adrenal glands and cortisol. What are adrenal glands and cortisol? Simply put, cortisol is one of the stress hormones. It is created by our adrenal glands (two small organs attached to our kidneys) and is mainly released during times of stress (Bunzenmeyer, personal communication, 2010). However, it also has many other important functions in your body. Having the right cortisol balance is essential for health. You can experience problems if you have too much or too little cortisol in your system.

In my case, according to Dr Bunzenmeyer, the issue was too much of it. Because my levels of stress and busyness had gone unchecked for so long, my adrenal glands were constantly being signalled to produce cortisol. I had no idea what my lifestyle was doing to my poor adrenals. They were working overtime and eventually got so tired that they "burned out." Suddenly, the glands that produce the hormones to regulate my body's stress responses, blood pressure, metabolism, sleep patterns, hormones, digestion, memory, and mood were no longer balancing properly. No wonder I was such a mess! What Dr Bunzenmeyer was explaining to me was something she referred to as "adrenal fatigue," also known as adrenal dysregulation, and she recommended we move forward with treatment based on that. Although not all physicians recognize "adrenal fatigue" as a medical condition, this diagnosis was very helpful to me, because it made me think about stress in a completely new way.

Stress made me sick? I had to adjust my thinking to understand this. At that time, I would never have described my life as stressful. Sure, I had a very full, busy life, but I had never tuned in to how I was feeling because I was so busy "doing stuff" all the time. I'm not suggesting that all stress is "bad" for us or that if you also have a busy, full life you will get sick the way I did. However, I am encouraging you to make sure you are regularly tuning in and being honest with yourself about how you are feeling physically and emotionally.

 For Indigenous Peoples, living on the land meant life flowed naturally. Daily life was moving with the cycles and rhythms of the land. The animals found in our territories were our teachers, and so we quickly learned the medicines gifted to us from the Earth and taught to us by the animals. In present times, Indigenous Peoples face many stressful situations every day. Stress is highly present in us as Indigenous People because of intergenerational trauma, which now presents itself as dis-ease.—*North Star*

What Is Stress for You?

In my work as a wellness facilitator over the past six years, I have discovered that the phrase "stressed out" has become a catch-all phrase that means different things to different people. One person might say they are stressed out when they are really busy, while another person says it when they are feeling anxious or worried.

Reflect and Respond
- What does the phrase "stressed out" mean to you?
- How does it show up in your body? For example, do you get headaches, clench your jaw, or experience tightness in your chest? Or maybe you have a hard time falling asleep or staying asleep? If you don't know the answer to this question, that is okay. Just start paying attention because it's an important thing to know about yourself.

- How do you react when you are feeling stressed out? Do you get quiet, lash out, or feel unusually emotional? If you don't know, ask someone you live or work with. They will be able to tell you!

Identifying your stress level and exploring how your body responds to it is strongly connected to mindfulness practices, as described in chapter 2, "Permission to Be Well." Being present and being mindful enables us to figure out our needs and then address our well-being accordingly.

Is All Stress Bad?

Is all stress bad? The short answer is no. Healthy levels of stress (eustresses) are motivating and energizing, and they can help us get stuff done. However, there is a point when stress can turn into a negative factor. When our stress levels are negatively affecting our physical and mental health, we know we have crossed the line. Zero stress isn't ideal either, because it can leave us feeling bored or unmotivated.

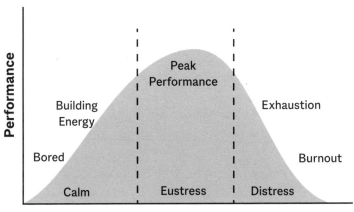

A Different Way to Think about Stress

I believe coping with negative stress is more about redefining our relationship with stress than it is about thinking we can eliminate it. Instead of just automatically reacting, it's more beneficial to focus on how we want to respond to negative stress when we experience it.

As Anishinaabe women, we gather once a month to receive teachings and spend time together. We receive teachings about the full moon and our connection to it. After we are finished sharing about the month we just experienced, we walk to the fire and sound our voices. We each sound our voices individually and then together as a group. The teaching behind this is that we let out our negativity and stress from the month we just completed by sounding our voices loudly to the moon. It is understood that after we sound our voices, we wait a second or two to take our first breath for the month ahead.—*North Star*

The Negative Stress Response

The stress response begins in the brain. According to Harvard Health (2020b), when our brain thinks we are in danger, a whole cascade of events starts taking place, including the following:

- "The amygdala sends a distress signal to the hypothalamus. This area of the brain functions like a command center, communicating with the rest of the body through the nervous system."
- Once the amygdala is triggered, the parts of the brain that help us with our executive functioning, memory, learning, creativity, and regulating our emotions shut down.
- The "hypothalamus activates the sympathetic nervous system by sending signals to the adrenal glands."
- The adrenal glands begin to produce cortisol and adrenalin. When we are facing a perceived danger, these help us prepare to fight, flee, or freeze (the response we often hear less about).

These are all good things to happen if we truly are in danger. The challenge is that our brain isn't great at determining what a real life-threatening situation is. It behaves the same way if we are reacting to a bolt of lightning (a real threat) as it does to looking at an overwhelmingly long to-do list (not a real threat).

Therefore, we need to have in-the-moment strategies so we can turn off that negative stress response when it isn't needed.

In-the-Moment Strategies

Fortunately, most people have end-of-the-day strategies to de-stress. Exercising, watching TV, reading, listening to music, and enjoying a hobby are common choices.

The problem, however, is if we wait only until the end of the day to deal with the stresses we feel, it's too late.

I'd like to challenge you to start thinking about what you do in the moment. When it's 9 am and you are already feeling anxious about the parent meeting coming up at noon, or when it's 1:30 pm and you are feeling overwhelmed by the staff meeting at the end of the day—what do you do then?

If we don't do something about it in the moment, then we will be under stress all day long. This can impair our health; it can also affect how we think and respond to events and people throughout the day.

Why Breathing Makes Sense

The great news is that there are many in-the-moment strategies we can use to turn off our stress response, and one of them is something we already do, all day, every day—*breathe.*

We've all heard the advice "take a deep breath" when it comes to dealing with stress. Some of you may have even rolled your eyes when you read that. There is, however, biological and neurological truth to the advice. When we take a long, slow, deep breath, the following happens:

- We activate the parasympathetic nervous system, which is responsible for our rest and relax response.
- The amygdala gets the message that our life isn't in danger, so it turns off. Once that happens, the other parts of the brain that were previously shut down come back online. Because of this, we can think more clearly.
- A message is also sent to our adrenal glands to stop producing cortisol and adrenalin. (Long, 2021)

All of that happens with the simple act of shifting how we breathe!

 As part of our Anishinaabe healing ceremonies, we looked at the Four Directions teachings of the Sacred Hoop to help us balance our healing. Breath is important when participating in a Sweat Lodge ceremony, when water medicine is poured on the heated rocks. As it gets hotter and hotter, we naturally breathe the hot medicine into our bodies, filling our lungs. This helps us regulate our breath into a more natural way of breathing, letting go of tension and inviting the healing in.—*North Star*

Stress-Busting Breathing Techniques

When we are feeling stressed, our breathing tends to be short, shallow, and irregular, so we want to shift it to a slower, deeper rhythm. But before you begin these breathing exercises, be mindful and present.

Find a comfortable position to sit in. One option is to position your feet flat on the ground and place your hands on your thighs to help ground you. Now, find an anchor. Maybe it is the breath itself, but it might also be an object or a sound. Anything that helps you anchor your attention to the present. Now you are ready to try these breathing strategies.

Here is a range of different breathing techniques to try. Please note that I did not create any of these. Rather, they are ones I have learned about over the years. Not every exercise will work for everyone. The goal is to experiment. Try them out and see what feels best for you. You may choose a couple—one you do in private and another that you can do when you are working or out in public. Choose something easy for you to remember and repeat and that feels effective for you. You can't get this wrong!

Three Slow, Gentle Deep Breaths

I love this one because it is so simple.

- Take three slow, gentle, deep breaths … whatever that means to you.
- If, after taking three, you feel like you need more, repeat!

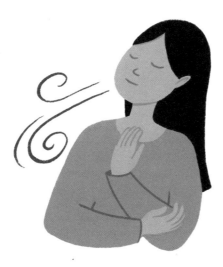

4-7-8 Breathing

Developed by Dr Andrew Weil (2016), this technique is powerful anytime, especially at night if you are having a hard time falling asleep.

1. Close your mouth and inhale deeply through your nose for a count of *four.*
2. Hold for *seven* counts.
3. Exhale slowly through your mouth for *eight* counts.
4. Breathe like this for *four* cycles, then return to "normal" breathing.

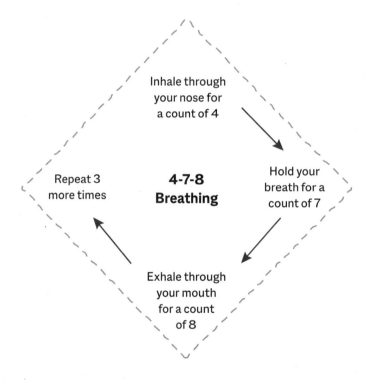

Rhythmic Breathing

As the name suggests, this technique is about getting your breath into a rhythm. Here are a few variations to try.

4–1–4

1. Breathe in through your nose for the count of *four.*
2. Hold for *one* count.
3. Exhale out your mouth for the count of *four.*
4. Repeat for at least two minutes.
5. If the count of four doesn't feel right to you, try 3–1–3 or 5–1–5. Just ensure your inhale and exhale are the same duration. Play with it to find what feels best for you.

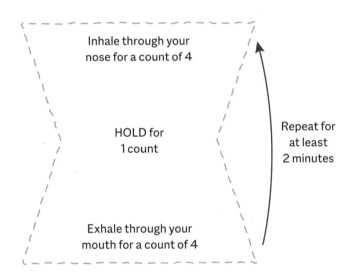

Inhale through your nose for a count of 4

HOLD for 1 count

Repeat for at least 2 minutes

Exhale through your mouth for a count of 4

Square Breathing, or Box Breathing
This technique, used by Navy SEALs to defuse stress, gets its name from the visual image used for counting as you breathe (Divine, 2016).

1. Inhale through your nose for a count of *four.*
2. Hold for a count of *four.*
3. Exhale through your mouth for a count of *four.*
4. Hold for a count of *four.*
5. Do this for as long as you need.

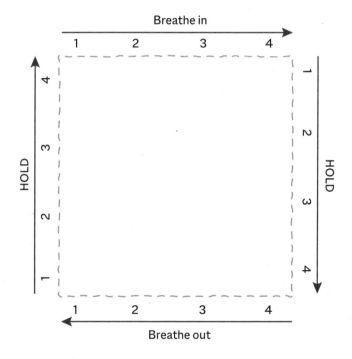

Hand Breathing

This is a great technique if you are a tactile person, as you may also enjoy the feeling of this one. It is also called Five-Finger Breathing.

1. Starting on the thumb side of your hand, inhale as you use your pointer finger on the other hand to trace upward along your thumb.
2. Exhale as you trace downward on the other side.
3. Repeat this pattern for the remaining four fingers.
4. Do this for as long as you need.

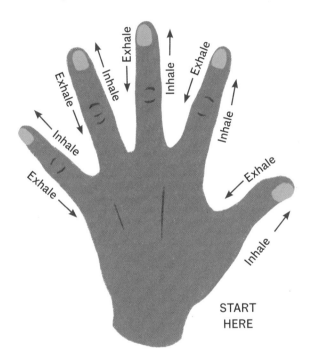

START
HERE

Alternate-Nostril Breathing

This one is my favourite. Alternate-nostril breathing originated thousands of years ago from the breath-control branch of yoga called pranayama (Urban, 2022). I always feel very calm and grounded after a few minutes of breathing like this.

1. Use your right thumb to seal your right nostril.
2. Inhale for a count of *four* through your left nostril, then seal the left nostril with your index finger.
3. Open the right nostril and exhale for a count of *six* through this side.
4. Inhale through the right nostril, then seal this nostril with your thumb.
5. Open the left nostril and exhale through the left side.
6. This is one cycle.
7. Continue for up to five minutes, or longer if it feels comfortable to do so.

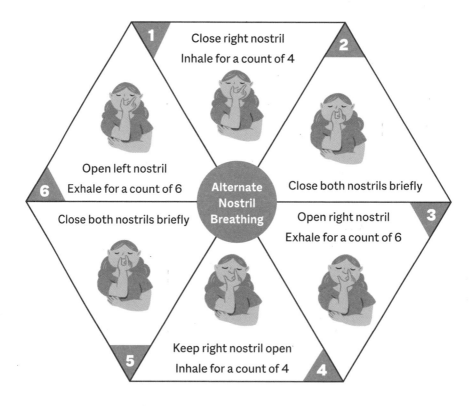

When my People go to the Tree of Life at the Sundance, we are worked on by a Healer. They usually work on us with their eagle bone whistles, and either breathe through the whistle to clear things away from our body or to suck our sickness out of us. This is using our breath to heal. This also occurs when we are smoking our pipes for healing. The breath of our prayers is the smoke from our pipe that makes its way back up to the Creator. We do similar breathing throughout many of our healing ceremonies. We are constantly reminded in our ceremonies that breath is sacred.—*North Star*

Twenty Minutes a Day

While deep breathing during moments of stress is important, there is growing consensus in the medical profession that we could benefit from spending at least 20 minutes each day doing some sort of deep breathing, regardless of how we are feeling (Hartley, 2020).

Why should we spend time deep breathing even when we are feeling good? It's the same reason why we practise fire drills at school—so if a real emergency happens, we know exactly what to do without having to think about it too much. When we regularly breathe deeply, it will become a practice that we can immediately use in times of stress. Another benefit is that, with regular practice, you can reset your stress thresholds. It takes time and consistency, but it is possible.

If 20 minutes per day seems like an impossible goal, know that it does not have to be 20 minutes all at once. You can do five minutes here and two minutes there, throughout the day. You'll be surprised how easy it can be to make the time when you are intentional about it.

To start, where can you find just a few minutes in your day to do some sort of deep breathing? Remember that the ultimate goal is 20 minutes per day, and even more on days when we are stressed out.

Closing Thoughts

It's been 11 years since my first appointment with the naturopath. What a journey it has been. Do I still get stressed out? Of course I do—I am human, after all. Do I still sometimes forget to take some deep breaths in the moment? Yup, but 80 percent of the time, I remember. At first, I couldn't imagine finding 20 minutes in my day to breathe deeply. But my health depended on it. Now, it's my go-to in-the-moment strategy for coping with stress. I also look forward to it on days when all is well. I can't imagine my life without it.

As you continue to read, pause and bring mindfulness to your breath. Breathe without judging whether your breathing is fast or even paced. Pick just one exercise that may help you as you continue your journey.

My heartfelt wish is that you will make the time to find a breathing technique that works for you so that you can experience all its benefits, including protecting and preserving your precious health.

> Feelings come and go like clouds in a windy sky.
> Conscious breathing is my anchor.
> —*Thich Nhat Hanh*

References and Further Reading

Ankrom, S. (2021). *8 deep breathing exercises to reduce anxiety*. Verywell mind. https://www.verywellmind.com/abdominal-breathing-2584115

Anxiety Canada. (n.d.). *Mindfulness exercises*. Retrieved May 1, 2021, from https://www.anxietycanada.com/articles/mindfulness-exercises/

Berryman, S. (2020). *Working well: Twelve simple strategies to manage stress and increase productivity*. Manage to Engage.

Dietz, K. (2021, November 5). *Try this quick technique to calm your anxiety*. Sharecare. https://www.sharecare.com/coronavirus/five-finger-breathing-anxiety

Divine, M. (2016, May 4). The breathing technique a Navy SEAL uses to stay calm and focused. *Time.* https://time.com/4316151/breathing-technique-navy-seal-calm-focused/

eMentalHealth.ca. (2021). *Deep breathing.* https://www.ementalhealth.ca/Canada/Deep-Breathing/index.php?m=article&ID=62559

Fletcher, J. (2019, February 12). How to use 4-7-8 breathing for anxiety. *Medical News Today.* https://www.medicalnewstoday.com/articles/324417#benefits

Gotter, A. (2020, June 17). Box breathing. *Healthline.* https://www.healthline.com/health/box-breathing#benefits

Hartley, A. (2020). *Breathe well: Easy and effective exercises to boost energy, feel calmer, more focused and productive.* Kyle Books.

Harvard Health. (2020a, July 6). Relaxation techniques: Breath control helps quell errant stress response. *Harvard Health Blog.* https://www.health.harvard.edu/mind-and-mood/relaxation-techniques-breath-control-helps-quell-errant-stress-response

———. (2020b, July 6). Understanding the stress response. *Harvard Health Blog.* https://www.health.harvard.edu/staying-healthy/understanding-the-stress-response

Long, C. (2021, August 30). *How the parasympathetic nervous system can lower stress.* HSS. https://www.hss.edu/article_parasympathetic-nervous-system.asp

Marksberry, K. (2012). *Take a deep breath.* AIS. https://www.stress.org/take-a-deep-breath

Mishler, A. (2014, January 22). *Yoga breathing / Alternate nostril breathing* [Video, 10:57]. YouTube. https://www.youtube.com/watch?v=8VwufJrUhic

Pizer, A. (2020, June 30). *Sama vritti pranayama for reducing stress.* Verywell fit. https://www.verywellfit.com/sama-vritti-equal-breathing-3566764

Scott, E. (2020, December 12). *Box breathing techniques and benefits.* Verywell mind. https://www.verywellmind.com/the-benefits-and-steps-of-box-breathing-4159900

Stinson, A. (2018, June 1). What is box breathing? *Medical News Today.* https://www.medicalnewstoday.com/articles/321805

Tocino-Smith, J. (2022, June 23). What is eustress and how is it different than stress? *Positive Psychology.* https://positivepsychology.com/what-is-eustress/

Urban, N. (2022, February 5). *9 scientific benefits of alternate nostril breathing.* Outliyr. https://outliyr.com/alternate-nostril-breathing-benefits

Weil, A. (2016, May). *Three breathing exercises and techniques.* https://www.drweil.com/health-wellness/body-mind-spirit/stress-anxiety/breathing-three-exercises/

Chapter 7

Finding Joy(ce)
My Journey from Burnout to Wisdom and Well-Being

Joyce Sunada

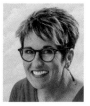

Joyce Sunada has more than 30 years of experience as an educator. During that time, she was a teacher, an administrator, and a provincial leader who helped create and support healthy school communities. She was also an instructor with the Werklund School of Education at the University of Calgary. Joyce offers educators one solid piece of advice: "If you don't take time for your wellness, you will be forced to take time for your illness." As Joyce now enters retirement, her most cherished role is being Jo Jo to her first grandchild, Deacon.

It was April 2006. I was an assistant principal in a parent meeting that was not going well. Tempers were rising, accusations were flying around the room, and my confidence was dwindling. As the meeting progressed, I remember checking out and thinking, "I didn't imagine my career in education would end like this!" Suddenly the door slammed shut—the parents had left the meeting. I crumpled onto the boardroom table and bawled as I had never bawled before.

My principal took me into her office, leaned over, and said, "Joyce, maybe you should take a break and go for a run." I took a deep breath and looked up at her. Even though this had been my go-to stress relief strategy, in my head I was thinking, "If I go for a run right now, it's going to be home to my basement, and I am never coming out again!"

How does an energetic and enthusiastic teacher end up feeling like a twisted, crumpled piece of metal in a train wreck? Quite simply, by not recognizing the signs that a train was coming down the track. This parent meeting was simply the straw that broke the camel's back. It was not the actual cause of my mental and emotional breakdown, but it was the tipping point that indicated burnout.[1]

What Is Burnout?

At the time of my "crash and burn," I'm not sure I used the term "burnout." Nor was I even aware that the word could describe my emotional and physical collapse, even though many people often casually speak of being burned out. The concept was originally described by Freudenberger (1975) and further explored by Maslach, Shaufeli, and Leiter (2009). More recently, Emily and Amelia Nagoski (2020) expanded our understanding of the issue. Burnout is defined as having three elements:

- Emotional exhaustion: the fatigue that comes from caring too much, for too long.
- Depersonalization: the depletion of empathy, caring, and compassion (sometimes referred to as cynicism).
- Decreased sense of efficacy and accomplishment: an unconquerable sense of futility, feeling that nothing you do makes a difference. (Adapted from Nagoski and Nagoski, 2020, p. xi)

Interestingly, recent research by these authors indicates that, for people in caring professions, like teachers, burnout is a significant mental health issue affecting up to 30 percent of us (Nagoski and Nagoski, 2020, p. xi).

So, if you are experiencing symptoms of burnout, you are not alone. What are those symptoms?

---

1   This chapter explores alternative therapies and treatments for wellness that may or may not be supported by medical science. These are based on the author's experiences, and are not intended as medical advice. Please check with a doctor before beginning any new treatment plan or making significant changes to your health-care routines.

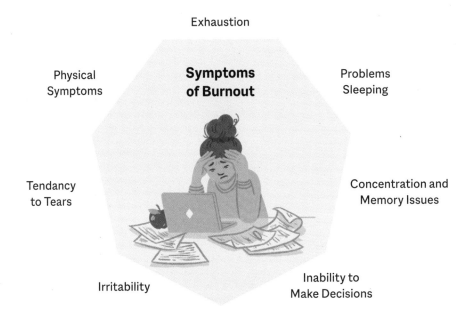

Exhaustion

Physical
Symptoms

**Symptoms
of Burnout**

Problems
Sleeping

Tendancy
to Tears

Concentration and
Memory Issues

Irritability

Inability to
Make Decisions

Perhaps, as a teacher, you can identify with some of the symptoms that I experienced. Maybe you:

- Wake up wondering how you will possibly get through the day
- Have frequent headaches and often feel run down
- Find yourself resentful or overwhelmed, even by a small request
- Avoid going to the staff room
- Eat on the go, alone, or while working
- Can't shut your mind off work
- Over-talk about work at home

Hindsight, as we know it, is very clear. I now see that I was experiencing many of the elements described here right before my crash. There were flags that I missed before I burned myself out.

Flag 1: Living at a Frenetic Pace

For a few years before and during the year I crashed, I was an assistant principal with teaching responsibilities at a one thousand-student elementary/junior high school. I was in constant fast-forward motion, firing on all cylinders to meet the demands of each day. I was speed-walking up and down the hallways of our school, pausing only to gulp oxygen in the middle of conversations, never able to catch my breath. In addition, I was experiencing annoying chest palpitations but chose to ignore them.

Flag 2: Lack of Self-Efficacy and Accomplishment

Constant battles were raging in my head. I accused myself of being an incompetent administrator, mother, and person. I thought that if I could just do more, accomplish more, I'd be worthy of the responsible position I held. Rather than strengthening me, this frenzied thinking rendered me powerless. I didn't believe I had the capacity. I felt that nothing I ever did made a difference.

Flag 3: Substantial Memory Loss and Difficulty Focusing

At that time, my husband and I were raising three daughters who all played high-level soccer. I was working full-time, volunteering with their teams when I could, and trying to enjoy my life. Having so many commitments taxed my brain. I frequently caught myself saying, "I'm not sure. I can't remember," and then laughing it off. At first, I found it humorous. Soon it became frustrating, then downright concerning. Often, I could not get from the front office to my own office, 20 steps away, without forgetting why I was heading there. On more than one occasion, I had to backtrack and ask my administrative assistant what I was going to do. I was grateful that she paid attention and could always help me out. When teachers made requests, I usually found myself having trouble focusing and remembering what to do next. My cognitive skills were being depleted as I began to burn out.

Flag 4: Continually Feeling Exhausted

My role as an administrator could have been empowering and exciting. But instead of feeling like I was making a difference, I felt an underlying tiredness most of the time. Being a former high-level athlete, farm kid, and energetic person, I would simply push through the fatigue. I wanted to look good and show staff, students, and parents that I was highly capable of performing my job. I would arrive at school with a big smile, hiding the weight I carried on my shoulders. Around 2 pm, I'd head to the canteen and purchase a sugary treat, having not made time to nourish myself well throughout the day. The boost of energy helped me make it to the end of the school day. I would trek home to get supper ready for my family and go to bed by about 8:30 pm. This exhaustion affected my family, as I didn't have the capacity to be present with them or help with their needs.

My illness also adversely affected my marriage. I experienced a lack of connection with my husband, which affected our communication and intimacy. Regardless of how or when he reached out, I was frequently disengaged and distracted. Our relationship became strained.

Flag 5: A Constant Feeling of Hopelessness

In my last year as an administrator, I had become quite despondent. Usually, we teachers come back to school in September excited, rested, and sun-kissed from our summer adventures. We are at low tide and the water level is at our ankles. We are anticipating the year, genuinely enjoying one another's company for the few days before the students arrive.

Once the students arrive, the water level rises a bit—as do our stress levels—until we settle our students into their daily routines. Later in the month comes Meet the Teacher Night, and the parents show up to check us out. Again, the water level rises, as we promise to provide the best education we can for their children. We are still feeling confident, energetic, positive, and mostly optimistic.

In a good year, the water levels ebb and flow like the tides. We face challenges, experience successes, complete report cards, survive parent-teacher interviews, coach teams, plan winter concerts, and then ease back into our comfortable routines.

In my last year as an administrator, the water levels never dropped. By spring, they had risen so high that I was concerned that if I stopped to take a breath, I would drown. But instead, I just kept swimming.

Until one day I found myself in a precarious situation. After another very long day at school, I drove home, pulled into the garage, and put the van in park. I let out a heavy sigh and was overwhelmed by thoughts: "I can't do this anymore. I could just end this. Then all of this—the frenetic pace, constant memory loss, exhaustion, and hopelessness—would be done."

I stumbled into the house and cried. It was one of the lowest moments of my life. I share it, not for your sympathy but rather to spark hope that we—you as well as I—can creep back into the light no matter how dark a situation becomes.

After that moment and the difficult parent meeting I described at the beginning of this chapter, I realized I needed a change. I decided to leave administration. I truly believed that being an assistant principal was the problem. Even then, I didn't notice the red flags. I concluded that it was the demands of my job that were causing the health issues in my life. I took a position at a small elementary school, hoping for a change in pace. Although I tried to enjoy my energetic Grade 5 class, I was totally out of my comfort zone. I quickly realized the stress level was just as high as it had been in administration. Once again, I was exhausted and crying on my way to and from work. And it was only September.

It was time to reach out for professional support. I had resisted before, but now I was ready. I was grateful for my employee benefits. They meant my employer cared about workplace wellness enough to acknowledge employees' psychological needs and address them at systems levels.

In early October, in a counselling session, I was diagnosed with depression. I was given a medical leave that would last nearly two years. This diagnosis was an "aha" moment for me to recognize the importance of self-care.

If you don't take time for your wellness, you will be forced to take time for your illness. Take some time now to think about wellness as it relates to your current role in education. Whether you are a seasoned veteran or new to the field of education, you can adapt the following reflections for your current situation. Any insight and awareness you gain now will serve you well over time. Be gentle with yourself. Don't dismiss the signs that something is not right. Notice them. If you are currently feeling well, you can still do this reflection proactively to establish a baseline and prevent burnout in the future.

Reflect and Respond

Pause now, put your feet flat on the floor, and take a few slow, deep, cleansing breaths. Relax. Be still and just breathe. When you feel calm, reflect on your past few months of teaching. Record anything that you are experiencing. Take note of things you would consider to be your red flags.

- What have you noticed about your behaviour, your feelings, and your ability to teach in the way you want to teach?
- How satisfied and joyful are you feeling about your teaching role?
- How's your energy level?
- Is there an action you can take to improve your situation? Is there someone you can reach out to for help?

My Journey to Wisdom and Wellness

I lived a great deal of my life thinking that I was not good enough. When I went on medical leave, my position was filled in three days. To me, that was a sign that I could be easily replaced by one of many eager and competent teachers lined up behind me.

Fortunately, we did not have money worries when I went on leave. For a long time, however, fear of the stigma of mental illness led me to avoid telling people why I was not working.

I had trouble believing that I was worthy of being taken care of, especially when it came to my well-being. I tried my best to take care of my family and friends, but putting myself first did not come naturally to me. I now know that when I practise self-care and focus on my overall health, I feel balanced and grounded. When I put my well-being first, I am better able to support others as well.

On my healing journey, I explored many non-conventional wellness experiences that have had a huge impact on my physical, emotional, mental, and spiritual health. I've discovered that each of us travels a very personal, courageous, and vulnerable path. It is something we do for ourselves, but it can require a great deal of outside support. Once we choose to embark on our healing path, the possibilities and supports present themselves. Know that your wellness journey is as unique as you are. Keep an open mind, but never feel that, because someone else has tried something, you need to do it, too. Trust yourself to know that you will identify the actions and people who can support you.

 As an Indigenous Person, I believe that our Healing Path or Journey is lifelong. We never consider ourselves well or healed. We know we must be constantly vigilant and mindful of our past and the need to continue to practise the good life. For us, a good life means living in harmony and balance. It means feeling well physically, emotionally, mentally, and spiritually.—*Elder Kipling*

Even while I participated in several non-conventional healing experiences, I also worked closely with the medical community and counsellors during my initial recovery from burnout. I found that choosing the professionals who could help me was not an either/or decision. Rather, I found different kinds of support from many. I embraced a holistic approach.

It has been 15 years since I burned myself out. I continue to experience ups and downs in all aspects of my life and my wellness. There is no end point. Gaining and maintaining a healthy existence is a lifelong adventure for all of us.

 I was taught by my Elders that when we are struggling, people, animals, and birds will come to us to provide support. We just need to be aware, prepared, and accepting of the help they are offering. The support is not always physical or even tangible. We call these Spirit Helpers and Guides sent by the Creator or the Ancestors.—*Elder Kipling*

The first step in my healing journey occurred the moment after my principal suggested that I go for a run. She picked up the phone and connected me to our district's counselling services. As hesitant as I was to take this action, I was eventually grateful. I didn't have the strength, courage, or knowledge on my own to access counselling at that time. When the counsellor identified that I was suffering from depression, I felt relieved. Now I had a diagnosis, and something could be done to help me. There are times when we need others to nudge, guide, and support us along the way, especially when we are unable to support ourselves.

I had a very close friend, my next-door neighbour, a retired teacher named Marilyn, who could see me struggling. As we walked our dogs each morning, she offered a kind heart and a listening ear. She was able to guide and support me, not only with her words but with her connections to the people who have supported me on my wellness journey. Marilyn suggested that I see her naturopath. Having someone take the time to regard me holistically was a new experience. This was one of the important steps I took as I began to regain my physical health.

Finding My Path

In my case, healing involved a range of modalities. In addition to counselling, I engaged in ThetaHealing, a form of meditation and spiritual philosophy. ThetaHealing helped me release many negative thoughts. I was able to engage my mind, body, and spirit: transforming limiting beliefs and working toward a positive lifestyle. I also used massage and worked with a Reiki master. Reiki is a traditional Japanese technique for stress reduction and relaxation that is believed to promote healing. There was no one "right" thing that I did. I was open and needed help, and I stuck with what was working for me. I also trusted the people whom I worked with along the way.

Learning to Journey

My road to wellness was also greatly influenced by working with a spiritual healer. She taught me how to "journey" so that I could tap into different realms to find wisdom and support (Daniels, 2020). In some traditions, journeying is believed to be a method of accessing information from what is called "non-ordinary reality" (Geddes, 2007, p. 3). This deep level of work further supported my healing. A lot of healing happened that I didn't even realize needed to take place. I gained more confidence and momentum to move forward.

Minding My Mindset

Throughout my healing journey, I learned about mindset. Depending on the messages we hear and choose to listen to, the mind can drive us to accomplish great feats, or it can bring us crumbling to our knees with fear and doubt.

For instance, I missed the first deadline to submit my chapter for this book project. I had convinced myself that I was an incompetent, inadequate imposter with little knowledge of wellness. These were hurtful thoughts that I would never say to anyone else. In the end, however, with self-awareness and self-compassion, I was able to believe in myself and move forward to complete this chapter. When I became aware of how I was speaking to myself about writing, I could work to reframe my self-talk. I could speak to myself more like I would to a dear friend. I also reached out for support and shared how I was struggling. These combined actions led to words of encouragement, hopefulness, and yes—writing my story!

Knowing how the mind works and having the ability to focus on what I can control has been transformative. I am not always optimistic, but I recognize that I can choose my thoughts, words, actions, habits, and values. We need to focus our energy on ourselves, reflect on our wellness, and practise self-care. This also means practising self-compassion and being kind to yourself on your journey. How you treat yourself has a direct impact on your wellness.

Reflect and Respond
- Are you treating yourself as you would your best friend?
- Take a close look at what you say to those individuals near and dear to you.
- When others mess up, do you chastise them or do you listen empathetically, offer support and reassurance, and forgive them?
- Put yourself in their shoes and treat yourself in the same compassionate way.

The Great Outdoors

I live a five-minute walk from Fish Creek Provincial Park in Calgary, Alberta, Canada. It is a wonderful natural area with a lovely flowing creek, thriving vegetation and wildlife, and kilometres of pathways you can bike and walk along. A feeling of aliveness emanates from the earth. During my medical leave, my relationship with Fish Creek deepened significantly. I had never considered the value or power of intentionally spending time connecting to the earth, being with the land.

Most of us enjoy spending time in nature. In fact, research shows that "spending at least 120 minutes a week in nature is associated with good health and wellbeing" (White et al., 2019). Interestingly, this study indicates that the pattern holds across age groups and regardless of other health conditions. Overall, being in nature is good for the whole person—physically, emotionally, mentally, and spiritually. A relatively new approach to nature-based wellness comes from Japan:

> We practice something called forest bathing, or *shinrin-yoku*. *Shinrin* in Japanese means "forest," and *yoku* means "bath." So *shinrin-yoku* means bathing in the forest atmosphere, or taking in the forest through our senses. This is not exercise, or hiking, or jogging. It is simply being in nature, connecting with it through our senses of sight, hearing, taste, smell and touch. *Shinrin-yoku* is like a bridge. By opening our senses, it bridges the gap between us and the natural world. (Li, 2018)

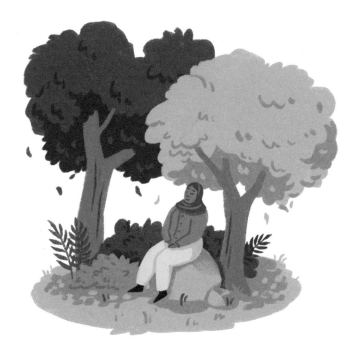

The research on forest bathing suggests that the benefits are both physiological and psychological, especially in reducing chronic stress (Hansen, Jones, and Tocchini, 2017).

When I needed it most, I was unconsciously drawn to the natural environment. I would sit or lie on the Earth and listen to the flowing water. I would gaze at the sky. I felt held, in a gentle and sustaining way. I would do this as often as I could. I came back home feeling rejuvenated, hopeful, and much less depressed.

The great outdoors continues to be a wellness anchor for me—I feel connected and strong. I have a sense of being nourished by the natural elements. I believe this relationship started when I was young on the farm in Cranford, Alberta. I am so grateful that I found it again.

 The land is where Indigenous People do the spiritual work that enables us to be well. We need to be on the land, talking to Mother Earth, harvesting the gifts from the land, such as preparing hides, feathers, bones, and plants. This is spiritual medicine given to us by the land, and this is what fosters wellness.—*Elder Kipling*

Closing Thoughts

If you are starting your career as an educator, I hope that you will stay connected to yourself. Notice red flags if they come up. Be open to what others share with you. Along the way, others who care about you may notice signs that you miss in yourself. If we listen, we can act early, bringing ourselves back on track.

If you are an experienced educator feeling that you are on a path to burnout, I hope you take good care of yourself. Treat yourself with loving kindness, as you would your own best friend. Realize it is possible to heal, and that your journey is unique to you. Trust yourself to lead you to the people, practices, and steps that will best serve you. Remember that your healing journey is unique to you, so honour it.

Reflect and Respond

Take a few minutes to reflect on the healing practices shared above.

- Do you already practise any of these healing modalities? Are there any new approaches to healing that have piqued your interest?
- Who would you consider asking for help on your wellness journey? Choose this person now, even if you are feeling perfectly well.
- Is there a traditional or non-traditional means of therapy that you know of and want to try?
- What action will you take as a result of reading this chapter?

References and Further Reading

Clay, R. (2018, February). Are you burned out? *CE Corner, 49*(2). https://www.apa.org/monitor/2018/02/ce-corner

Daniels, J. (2020). *About Jaki.* https://www.jakidaniels.com/aboutjaki

Freudenberger, H. J. (1975). The staff burn-out syndrome in alternative institutions. *Psychotherapy: Theory, Research & Practice, 12*(1), 73–82. https://doi.org/10.1037/h0086411

Geddes, M. (2007). *Ask the very beasts: Words of wisdom and comfort from unexpected sources.* Rattlesnake Books.

Hansen, M., Jones, R., & Tocchini, K. (2017). Shinrin-yoku (forest bathing) and nature therapy: A state-of-the-art review. *International Journal of Environmental Research and Public Health, 14*(8), 851. https://doi.org/10.3390/ijerph14080851

Li, Q. (2018, May 1). "Forest bathing" is great for your health. Here's how to do it. *Time.* https://time.com/5259602/japanese-forest-bathing/

Nagoski, E., & Nagoski, A. (2020). *Burnout: The secret to unlocking the stress cycle.* Ballantine Books.

Schaufeli, W. B., Leiter, M., & Maslach, C. (2009, June 19). Burnout: 35 Years of research and practice. *Career Development International, 14*(3), 204–20. doi:10.1108/13620430910966406

White, M., Alcock, I., Grellier, J., Wheeler, B., Hartig, T., Warber, S., Bone, A., Depledge, M., & Fleming, L. (2019, June 13). Spending at least 120 minutes a week in nature is associated with good health and wellbeing. *Scientific Reports, 9*(7730). https://doi.org/10.1038/s41598-019-44097-3

Chapter 8

Building Relationships for Well-Being

Jennifer E. Lawson with Shannon Gander,
Lisa Dumas Neufeld, and Kelsey McDonald

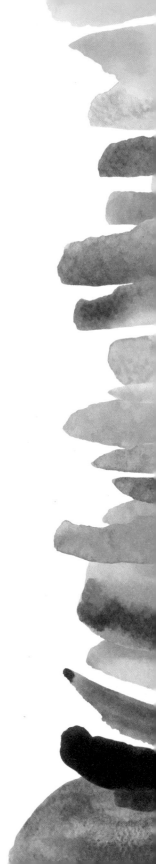

> I define connection as the energy that exists
> between people when they feel seen, heard, and valued;
> when they can give and receive without judgment;
> and when they derive sustenance and
> strength from the relationship.
> —*Brené Brown*

After just a few years of experience, I felt I had honed my craft in the classroom. I had taught in two rural school divisions in Manitoba and considered myself a master teacher. But then I got a new position in the inner city. I quickly realized that I was a total rookie when it came to meeting the needs of children and families in this community. My confidence declined and I felt unequipped for the role.

Fortunately, I soon discovered that I had been given the gift of a school culture of collegiality and support. There I experienced genuine connection, trust, and teamwork. It was a challenging school, but the staff felt a strong sense of purpose that we were doing more than teaching a curriculum. We were changing lives and, at times, even saving lives.

Adding to this were the personal connections. The staff worked hard, but we played hard as well. In such a challenging workplace, it wasn't uncommon for staff to cry, but there was often as much laughter as there were tears. We savoured moments of joy and success and socialized together often. Interestingly, there was a rule among staff that we were not allowed to talk shop during social events. If we did, we had to throw a loonie in the kitty for a food hamper for a local family. Our donations to the community grew at first but eventually, people learned to let go of difficult issues at work and simply share happiness. This had the added benefit that spouses and guests who attended social events felt much more part of the group because there was no teacher talk. The social connection on this staff was so strong that, even years after I and others had left the school, we still gathered annually to share that joy and sense of community.

There is no doubt that Brené Brown's definition of connection, which this chapter begins with, rang true for me in this school. I felt seen, heard, and valued, and I derived sustenance and strength from the relationships fostered there. The research on workplace wellness supports this idea. Collegial support is critical to fostering a positive work environment. The more employees feel they have this support, the greater their sense of workplace well-being, job satisfaction, and job performance (Guarding Minds at Work, 2020).

In this chapter we examine why and how good collegial relationships have been important to us as educators. We look at what experts say about high-quality connections and well-being and offer practical ways for teachers to build and maintain good relationships with colleagues. The tools and concepts are relevant across all relationships and interactions we hold as educators, both personal and professional.

Relationships are crucial to our development and well-being. Relationships have the power to cause pain and suffering, but they also have the power to heal and give new life.

The PERMAH model of well-being was introduced in chapter 2, "Permission to Be Well." Each element of the model offers a building block of well-being. I believe that the *R*, which stands for Relationships, is the foundation.

Relationships play a key role in almost all careers. That said, teaching is its own unique unicorn when it comes to relationships. We might be interacting with 20-plus adults and more than 100 children or youth in a single day. Whatever relational dynamics exist in our personal lives, we are continually navigating our own emotions alongside those of others.

Reflect and Respond

Think of a time when you experienced a positive relational community at work, one in which you felt seen, heard, and valued, when you had opportunities to give and receive without judgment, and gained energy and strength from your colleagues.

- What image or memory comes to mind?
- Who was there? Why was it energizing?
- How did you contribute to this energy and community?

Communities are built on strong natural bonds and relationships with the natural world. This is the foundation of Indigenous communities. The building and maintaining of our relationships can be found in Pipe Ceremonies and how we honour the Seven Sacred Teachings: Wisdom, Love, Respect, Bravery, Honesty, Humility, and Truth. The land and water speak to the strong natural bonds we have when they are at the centre of our prayers. We see our relationships as a circle, like the Sacred Hoop. You get a gift from the land, and you give a gift back to the land. This keeps us connected and committed.

Supportive and caring relationships are ingrained in an Indigenous perspective. If any member of the community was suffering or in need, the community would step up and help the family in need. If children in a community are orphaned, they are automatically adopted and welcomed into a family, and not seen as outsiders. This is why, today, you often hear people in our communities being called Aunty or Uncle when there is no blood relation. These close relationships reflect honour and respect for community members.—*North Star*

High-Quality Connections

High-quality connections (HQCs) are the connections of mutual trust, energy, positive regard, responsiveness, and respectful engagement made between two people. In a social ecosystem like a school, HQCs can be considered the life-giving oxygen that nourishes the people and practices within it (Fulwiler, 2019). HQCs generate a mutual energy that enriches us so much more than connections that simply "go through the motions of communication" (Dutton and Heaphy, 2003). Low-quality connections, which often consist of passive small talk, venting, and negative commentary, can be draining. In schools, we connect with people all day, every day. Even a brief interaction can be an HQC, which can provide a well-being boost and create a positive ripple effect.

Reflect and Respond
- Think of an energizing interaction you've recently had. It could be with someone you've known for a while or someone you just met.
- What was it about the interaction that left you feeling energized? What did you contribute to the exchange?

Research shows compelling benefits from building HQCs to enhance workplace wellness. HQCs can broaden our thinking and enhance our self-image. They can increase adaptability, cooperation, job satisfaction and commitment, and organizational citizenship (Dutton, 2019). Studies even show beneficial physiological effects of social interactions at work, including strengthening our immune system capacity (Heaphy and Dutton, 2008). HQCs can also build creativity, resilience, authenticity, and learning outcomes (Dutton and Heaphy, 2003; Dutton, 2019).

According to Jane Dutton (n.d.), we can intentionally cultivate HQCs using powerful questions. The questions are "powerful" because they foster positive connection and demonstrate authentic interest. Here are some examples of questions you can ask your colleagues that provide opportunities to convey genuine interest, explore support, or uncover common ground:

- What makes you feel valued here?
- What are the things others have done for you at work that you've found most helpful?
- Are there ways we could work together to lighten your load right now?
- What brings you joy outside of school?
- How do you rejuvenate during the summer months?

Try formulating your own powerful questions that relate to your coworkers and take the time to actively listen to their responses.

Relational Crafting

How can we build more opportunities for each other to be seen, heard, and valued? To give and receive without judgment, and allow ourselves and each other to be strengthened by our relationships?

 A Talking Circle is a valuable way for all community members to be seen, heard, and valued. It allows everyone to share their voice if they want to. As well, Indigenous forms of government allow all members of the community to have input, again suggesting that everyone's ideas are valuable. When this occurs, it strengthens relationships.—*North Star*

We make decisions all day, every day, about how we interact with our job. These choices affect our experience at work and how we feel about it. Organizational psychologists call this "job crafting" (Wrzesniewski and Dutton, 2001). Job crafting is happening all day, whether we are intentional about it or not. Job design is the top-down, external element that determines the courses and grades we teach, what our timetable is, when the bells will ring, and so on. Job crafting, on the other hand, is bottom-up. It describes how we customize our days. It involves the choices we make about who we interact with and how, if we mark during our preps or before or after school, and so on.

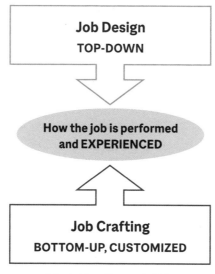

Adapted from Berg et al., 2013

Job crafting has been shown to enhance teachers' perception of meaningful work and to positively correlate with teacher resilience (Van Den Heuvel et al., 2015). It increases teachers' job satisfaction and engagement (Alonso et al., 2019) and supports early-career teachers with stronger job attachment and satisfaction (Leana et al., 2009).

"Relational crafting" is an important part of job crafting. This involves being intentional in how we think about the nature of our daily interactions with others (Berg et al., 2013). One example of an effective strategy for relational crafting is the practice of "savouring." Savouring means focusing our attention on moments in our day that fill us up and seeing things from a positive perspective to experience more pleasure (Hughes 2019).

For example, Lisa was sitting across the table from a very charismatic and frustrated 10-year-old. She was laying down some new classroom boundaries when he stood, picked up the chair by its metal leg, and threw it at the window. Lisa's first thought was, "Huh. I guess we do have a good relationship. He could have thrown it at me instead of the window."

Lisa had spent time connecting and savouring beautiful moments with him—on the floor doing sit-ups and lunges together for his afternoon movement break, helping him run a small "Magic Club" over recess, and sharing a love for the book *James and the Giant Peach*. These tiny moments were building a high-quality connection underneath his, and sometimes Lisa's own, dysregulation. The process of savouring the good has helped Lisa to reshape her thinking about students (and parents and colleagues) who struggle.

Intentionally building relationships at work is another strategy. For example, when Kelsey was a first-year teacher she struggled immensely, as you will read about in chapter 11, "Thank You for Being a Friend." One way she tried to manage was to work through lunch alone in her classroom. She thought if she just pushed herself hard enough, eventually she would feel on top of things. Fortunately for her, Kelsey's classroom neighbour Michelle was an observant and compassionate teacher who knew social isolation was not going to help. One day Michelle popped into Kelsey's classroom and invited her to take a walk for a change of scenery over the lunch hour. Over time, they built a friendship. Michelle encouraged Kelsey to join the staff room for lunch occasionally, intentionally crafting relationships with other colleagues. Kelsey found the right combination in a balance between time socializing with other staff, those one-on-one walks, and some days working on her own in her classroom.

These two examples demonstrate how we can enrich our daily practice with energizing experiences that enhance our well-being and contribute to the well-being of our peers. We have more control over our experience of our jobs than we might initially realize. We certainly have control over how we interact with others. Prioritizing energizing connections is empowering.

> **Reflect and Respond**
> Picture one of the most energizing experiences in your work life that contributes to your well-being.
> - What exactly is it about that experience that makes it so energizing?
> - What do you contribute?
> - What do other people contribute?
> - How might you "craft" more energizing interactions into your daily life at work?

Building on the Positive

Here are some strategies to help intentionally craft interactions and relationships that boost rather than drain our well-being. Active-constructive responding (ACR) is a dynamic, authentic, positive way of responding to others' good news (Gable and Reis, 2010; Gable et al., 2004). Instead of destructive or passive responses, you choose to purposely respond in an active-constructive way.

Consider this scenario. You share with a colleague that you just received a glowing note of thanks from a parent whose child had been struggling in math and was now making significant progress. You tell this colleague how much the note means to you because both you and the student worked hard to help them succeed.

An active-destructive response from this colleague might be, "Well, she's obviously hoping that her child gets a good grade and that's why she sent the note." This response may create a negative experience for you because it takes away from the parent's honourable and authentic intention.

An active-constructive response, in contrast, helps you celebrate your positive experience, reinforcing the feeling (Gable and Reis, 2010; Gable et al., 2004). For example, if your colleague says, "Wow, that's terrific. I bet you feel great getting a note like that from a parent, especially after all the work you have done to help their child. How are you feeling about it? Does it warm your heart?"

The intent of ACR is to help a person share and savour a positive experience and therefore benefit in their well-being. By being positive and interested in what they have shared, you are building on the positive for them and even for yourself.

This chart presents examples of various responses. Notice your automatic responses to others' good news and remember to intentionally work on active-constructive responses.

Responding to Someone Else's Good News		
	Active	Passive
Constructive	"Wow, that's great! How do you feel?" Enthusiastic support Eye contact Authentic	"That's nice. Good for you." Low energy Delayed response Quiet
Destructive	"Well, that sounds unlikely." Quashing the event Dismissive Demeaning	"Sorry, I'm busy—have to run." Turns focus inward Avoiding Ignores speaker

Source: Adapted from GoStrengths

We don't intend to respond in a destructive way when others share good news. Often, we're just trying to relate to them. Or our negativity bias leads us to naturally highlight the potential problems or dangers. Therefore, we need to be intentional with our responses to our colleagues. We need to park any urge to compare ourselves or thoughts that somehow their experience takes away from ours. Next time someone shares good news, pause and consider: How can I respond actively and constructively and help them capitalize on the well-being boost they're experiencing?

When Conflict Arises

There is no question that, even if we all work hard to build positive relationships, conflicts are going to arise in our personal and professional lives. The "drama triangle" (Karpman, [1968] 2020) has been a valuable tool used for years to help people explore their interpersonal relationships and how they navigate conflict. This model can make us more aware of the reactions we sometimes have to challenging events in our daily life that can affect our relationships.

When we are caught in the drama triangle, it can take a toll on our energy because conflict and disharmony in relationships can be both frustrating and exhausting. When there is drama within our staff teams, it can ripple beyond the individuals involved and negatively affect the wider team. Likely, we have all been a part of drama triangles, but we can work on developing more awareness of our habits and healthier ways of reacting. The key is to not get stuck in the triangle and have it be the only way you know how to handle conflict.

Look at the diagram below. The three points on the triangle represent three ways of reacting to conflict—responses that are more likely to prolong disharmony than end it. Below are descriptions of each position.

Drama Triangle

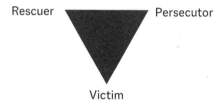

Rescuer: This position is often represented by the thought, "I am only okay if you are okay." It is very common among individuals who work in helping professions. As teachers, we want our students and colleagues to be okay. But if that means we can only feel peace and contentment when those around us are also at peace, it affects our well-being. Karpman (2020) suggests that rescuers may tend to apply short-term repairs to a victim's problems while neglecting their own needs. What that can mean for teachers who are in rescuer mode is that they expend so much energy supporting others that they can become stuck in a space of martyrdom (and impending burnout). This can have a significant impact on well-being.

Persecutor: This position is marked by the thought "I am okay, and you are the problem." Persecutors blame victims and criticize the enabling behaviour of rescuers. However, they tend not to provide guidance, assistance, or a solution to the underlying problem. At the same time, they often feel internally insecure and inadequate. Imagine, for example, that the school staff has been exploring a new curricular resource to use with students. A person in a persecutor position may resist and criticize this initiative. They may blame the person who came up with the idea and criticize others who support it. The truth may be, however, that the persecutor is afraid of change and does not feel confident about implementing the new resource. The underlying concern may be a feeling of self-doubt.

Victim: This position is marked by the thought "I am not okay, but I have done nothing wrong." A person in the victim position may blame someone else for the problem and, like the persecutor, may not try to help solve the problem. They might also look for a rescuer to save them. A teacher with an especially difficult class might feel like a victim for having more than their share of challenging students. They may blame their principal for the class makeup and not look for solutions within the learning environment.

Note that the victim position is not the same as being victimized or bullied during a specific event. In the drama triangle, assuming the victim position is more of an ongoing way of thinking of oneself during conflict. Most people, once they become aware of the positions of rescuer, persecutor, and victim, can see how they assume those positions in both their professional and personal lives.

Reflect and Respond
Think about when you might have taken on any of the positions of the drama triangle: rescuer, persecutor, or victim. Take the time to observe both the personal and professional areas of your life. Remember to do this with curiosity and without judgment. This is an awareness exercise.

You might be thinking to yourself, "Sure, I can acknowledge that sometimes I get drawn into the _____ position, but it's really hard to get out of it and do something different." Here are some strategies for each position that can help you mindfully remove yourself from the drama triangle.

If you find yourself in the "rescuer" position, your job is to notice and feel your own emotions. Those who are prone to rescuing have a low tolerance for witnessing the suffering and pain of others. Also, helping others makes us feel better about ourselves. When we see someone struggling, it can remind us of our insecurities and struggles, and we respond by rescuing that person. This also tends to keep the victim dependent on the rescuer. Slow down and reflect on the following questions. What is it about watching this person struggle that is so hard for me? What thoughts, beliefs, and emotions does this trigger for me and how can I manage them? Am I willing to step out of the rescuer position to allow others to work through their conflict?

If you find yourself in the "persecutor" position, your job is to put yourself in the other person's shoes and find some perspective. Even if you have to dig deep, find the good intentions of whoever or whatever you feel compelled to "persecute." Locate that place in your heart that has compassion for others. Activate your sense of empathy and recall times when you were not at your best and needed grace from yourself and others. Then, speak from there and act from there.

If you find yourself in the "victim" position, your job is to find one small thing to do. Those who see themselves as victims often render themselves helpless and powerless—a paralyzing position. You may truly be exhausted, struggling, and feeling a lack of support. The first step to getting out of the drama triangle when you are in this position is to *do* something. Act! You will be surprised at how empowered you begin to feel when you take a small action.

Conflict in the workplace is not just personally challenging. It also affects our ability to do our best work and to support collective well-being. We need to be aware of our behaviours and our responses to the behaviour of others. When we are self-aware, we are better able to address conflict situations, create more positive relationships, and promote workplace wellness.

An Indigenous Perspective on Healing Relations

I love the river … watching it, smelling it, looking at the light on it. I sit there with the plants, grasses, and insects, the mud, clay, bird bones, and shells. There's a resident eagle, pelicans, graffiti, geese, and the occasional abandoned shopping cart. There's also a crew of swallows that lives under the bridge; at dawn, they fly around in these mesmerizing formations. All these things create the whole. They're integrated, the mess and the magnificence.

Me, too. There are parts of me that are messy, and aspects that are exquisite. Once I become aware of what's there, I can begin to work with the different parts. My goal isn't to throw parts of myself *out* of the circle, but to get to know them and integrate them *into* the circle, something like the way we soothe and ease a wayward student into the school community. Thich Nhat Hanh (1992) has a practice for dealing with the messy, misguided parts of ourselves. We imagine that we are holding it … softly. We say something like, "Oh, hey, persecutor. I see you. I'll take care of you." With this gentle acknowledgement, transformation begins.

We can train ourselves to perceive the rescuer, persecutor, and victim as misguided aspects of ourselves and others. We are just hanging out, unskillfully trying to meet needs, in need of teaching and healing.

I was student-teaching at a youth centre and staff found a shank made of chicken bone in a young man's cell. He brought the bone back from lunch and shaved it down on the brick walls of his cell. I realized that this was divergent thinking, however misguided. Likewise, when we're acting out drama-triangle patterns, we can find the energy of skillful traits underneath. Under the pointed energy of a persecutor is a fierce advocate. Within the rescuer, there's a skilled facilitator. Within the victim, there is a very real tenderness.

In chapter 3, "Making Sense of Mindfulness," Keith Macpherson quotes Wayne Dyer (2009) who puts it this way: "When you change the way you look at things, the things you look at change."

Comparing Indigenous community healing to Western criminal justice, Rupert Ross noted that "Probably one of the most serious gaps in the system is the different perception of wrongdoing and how to best treat it. In the non-Indian community committing a crime seems to mean that the individual is a bad person and therefore must be punished … the Indian communities view a wrongdoing as a misbehaviour which requires teaching or an illness which requires healing" (2006).

Healing Circles are spaces that gather people: the offender, victim, families, and community. The offender speaks about their "personal healing journey in a way that touches on how they dealt with the underlying factors that led them to [act out] in the first place" (Chartrand and Horn, 2016). The victim shares how the incident has affected their lives in different dimensions. The families of both sides also share, and recommendations are made for reconciliation.

In chapter 4, "Restoring the Circle," I share a path to healing with the six *R*'s of my Integrated Reconciliation Framework model. One of the *R*'s is Relationships. As we cultivate the unskillful aspects of ourselves, our relationships are transformed. We can then, in time, guide others to heal and shift as well. But we can't authentically take anyone anywhere we haven't gone. We use what we have—grasses, shopping carts, glimmering shells, swallows, and all—and fold it into our Sacred Circle. There, we become deeply connected. Whole. Able to become servant-leaders.—*Lisa Dumas Neufeld*

Repairing After a Rupture

Ring the bells that still can ring
Forget your perfect offering
There is a crack in everything
That's how the light gets in
—*Leonard Cohen, "Anthem"*

Conflict is part of healthy relationships and is really an attempt at collaboration. Sometimes—because we are human—we might say something to a colleague, or someone else in our lives, and walk away feeling a little inner cringe. You know that feeling when you didn't like your tone or wished you had said something different. Maybe you were rushed, or you weren't quite at your best. You might have felt it both during the moment and after, upon reflection.

A relationship rupture is when we say or do something that can potentially injure a relationship. It's not uncommon to fall into the pattern of convincing ourselves that there is no point in revisiting the event after a rupture. We tell ourselves that it will feel awkward for the other person. We might feel silly or convince ourselves that the other person is probably mad and won't want to hear us out. So, we leave it. We may even pretend that nothing happened or avoid the other person for a while. That might lead to a second rupture when they wonder why we are mad at them.

Tammy Lenski has been a leader in conflict resolution and mediation since the early 1990s. Lenski shares a path to repair after a relationship rupture (2014). She borrows from author-activist Anne Lamott, who maintains that when we write, we are often willing to be vulnerable. We will pass our "lousy first draft" over to a friend or colleague, asking if they can work with it and make it better. In the case of our conversations, however, we tend not to do this. We are often unwilling to see the first interaction as only a first attempt. Lenski suggests that we allow ourselves a do-over after the lousy first draft conversation. Essentially, we give ourselves permission to go back and say to the other person what we wish we had said the first time.

Ruptures are inevitable. They are also often repairable. It does, however, take the ability to suspend our blame—of ourselves or the other person—and replace it with something more functional. We can all benefit from the do-over to the lousy first draft conversation. Not only does it go a long way toward repairing a potential relationship rupture but it also demonstrates care for the relationship. It shows that we want to try again. It's also great mentoring for healthy relationships in all areas of our life. We just have to be willing.

Reflect and Respond
- Consider whether you have experienced a lousy first draft conversation between you and someone you care about that would benefit from a do-over.
- What if you practised the do-over? Write what you would want to say to this person.
- Consider if you want to take the next step.

 The clans of the Anishinaabe were one way our People dealt with conflict. Our leadership clans were the Crane and the Loon Clan, and if they were unable to resolve a dispute or disagreement, they would go seek counsel with the Fish/Turtle Clan to help them solve the stalemate. If, for some reason, the conflict was not resolved, then other clans would be added to the mix until every clan in the community had a hand in resolving the issue. Today, some of our communities use the clan framework to help them with judicial practices, known as restorative justice, in the community.—*North Star*

Closing Thoughts

We are hardwired to connect. What those connections look, sound, and feel like is up to each of us. On any given day in teaching, we navigate relationships with colleagues, administration, students, parents, the public, community partners, our families, and ourselves. Those are a lot of different humans that we have the potential to have an impact on, and who can have an impact on us. How can we strengthen those connections?

Our relationships are built-in resilience resources that we can all access in times of struggle and triumph—especially when we realize the roles we each play in strengthening them.

Reflect and Respond

Think about your current workplace.

- Visualize and savour some of the positive relationships you have there.
- How have you created high-quality connections?
- How can you continue to build those kinds of connections with others? How might this affect you and your work environment?

 Indigenous teachings suggest that we are first born into a community and then to individuality afterward. We first have a responsibility to the well-being of the community, which in turn will seek to support the individual. It is only then that we will be able to think outwardly about the health and wellness of our territories and then the world.—*North Star*

References and Further Reading

Alonso, C., Fernández-Salinero, S., & Topa, G. (2019). The impact of both individual and collaborative job crafting on Spanish teachers' wellbeing. *Education Sciences*, *9*(2), 74. https://doi.org/10.3390/educsci9020074

Berg, J. M., Dutton, J. E., & Wrzesniewski, A. (2008, August 1). *What is job crafting and why does it matter?* University of Michigan, Ross School of Business, Center for Positive Organizational Scholarship. https://positiveorgs.bus.umich.edu/wp-content/uploads/What-is-Job-Crafting-and-Why-Does-it-Matter1.pdf

———. (2010, August 20). *Teaching note: Job crafting exercise.* University of Michigan, Ross School of Business, Center for Positive Organizational Scholarship. https://positiveorgs.bus.umich.edu/wp-content/uploads/Job-Crafting-Exercise-Teaching-Note-Aug-101.pdf

———. (2013). Job crafting and meaningful work. In B. J. Dik, Z. S. Byrne, & M. F. Steger (Eds.), *Purpose and meaning in the workplace* (pp. 81–104). American Psychological Association. https://doi.org/10.1037/14183-005

Brown, B. (2013). *Daring greatly: How the courage to be vulnerable transforms the way we live, love, parent and lead.* Portfolio Penguin.

Centers for Disease Control and Prevention. (2021). *Violence prevention: Adverse childhood experiences.* https://www.cdc.gov/violenceprevention/aces/index.html

Chartrand, L., & Horn, K. (2016). *A report on the relationship between restorative justice and Indigenous legal traditions in Canada.* Department of Justice Canada. https://www.justice.gc.ca/eng/rp-pr/jr/rjilt-jrtja/rjilt-jrtja.pdf

Doney, L., & Fulwiler, D. (2021). Crafting relational wellbeing [Unpublished manuscript].

Dutton, J. E. (n.d.). What questions work for you in building high quality connections? *WorkTies*. Retrieved September 1, 2021, from https://www.workties.org/post/what-questions-work-for-you-in-building-high-quality-connections

———. (2019, March 29). High quality connections: A keystone to positive institutions [PowerPoint presentation]. University of Michigan.

Dutton, J. E., and Heaphy, E. D. (2003). The power of high-quality connections. In K. S. Cameron, J. E. Dutton, & R. E. Quinn (Eds.), *Positive organizational scholarship: Foundations of a new discipline* (pp. 263–78). Berrett-Koehler.

Dyer, W. (2009). Success secrets. *Dr. Wayne W. Dyer.* https://www.drwaynedyer.com/blog/success-secrets/

Fulwiler, Dana. (2019). Infusing well-being into public education: A case for living it. (Publication Number 179) [Master of Applied Positive Psychology (MAPP) Capstone Project, University of Pennsylvania]. Scholarly Commons. https://repository.upenn.edu/mapp_capstone/179

Gable, S. L., Gonzaga, G. C., & Strachman, A. (2006). Will you be there for me when things go right? Supportive responses to positive event disclosures. *Journal of Personality and Social Psychology, 91*(5), 904–17. https://doi.org/10.1037/0022-3514.91.5.904

Gable, S. L., & Reis, H. T. (2010). Good news! Capitalizing on positive events in an interpersonal context. *Advances in Experimental Social Psychology, 42*, 195–257. https://doi.org/10.1016/S0065-2601(10)42004-3

Gable, S. L., Reis, H. T., Impett, E. A., & Asher, E. R. (2004). What do you do when things go right? The intrapersonal and interpersonal benefits of sharing positive events. *Journal of Personality and Social Psychology, 87*(2), 228–45. https://doi.org/10.1037/0022-3514.87.2.228

GoStrengths. (n.d.). *What is active and constructive responding?* Retrieved May 1, 2021, from https://gostrengths.com/what-is-active-and-constructive-responding/

Guarding Minds at Work. (2020). *Know the psychosocial factors.* https://www.guardingmindsatwork.ca/about/about-psychosocial-factors

Hanh, T. (1992). *Peace is every step: The path of mindfulness in everyday life.* Bantam Books.

Heaphy, E. D., & Dutton, J. E. (2008). Positive social interactions and the human body at work: Linking organizations and physiology. *Academy of Management Review, 33*(1), 137–62. https://psycnet.apa.org/record/2008-00018-008

Hughes, D. (2019, January 8). Is savouring the key to happiness at work? *Association for Talent Development.* https://www.td.org/insights/is-savoring-the-key-to-happiness-at-work

Karpman, S. B. (2020). The drama triangle. *Transactional Analysis Bulletin, 7*(26), 39–43. (Original article published in 1968 as "Fairy tales and script drama analysis.") https://karpmandramatriangle.com/

Leana, C., Appelbaum, E., & Schevchuk, I. (2009). Work process and quality of care in early childhood education: The role of job crafting. *Academy of Management Journal, 52,* 1169–92. https://doi.org/10.5465/amj.2009.47084651

Lenski, T. (2014, August 5). Sh**ty first drafts of difficult conversations. https://tammylenski.com/?s=first+draft

Tippet, K. (Host). (2016, September 22). Parker Palmer + Courtney Martin: The inner life of rebellion [Audio podcast episode]. In *On being.* https://onbeing.org/programs/parker-palmer-courtney-martin-the-inner-life-of-rebellion/

Perry, B. D. (2014, December 11). *Bruce D. Perry: Social and emotional development in early childhood* [Video, 1:00:27]. YouTube. https://www.youtube.com/watch?v=vkJwFRAwDNE

Reis, H. T., Smith, S. M., Carmichael, C. L., Caprariello, P. A., Tsai, F., Rodrigues, A., & Maniaci, M. R. (2010). Are you happy for me? How sharing positive events with others provides personal and interpersonal benefits. *Journal of Personality and Social Psychology, 99*(2), 311–29. doi:10.1037/a0018344

Ross, R. (2006). *Dancing with a ghost: Exploring Aboriginal reality.* Penguin Canada.

Van Den Heuvel, M., Demerouti, E., & Peeters, M. C. W. (2015). The job crafting intervention: Effects on job resources, self-efficacy, and affective well-being. *Journal of Occupational and Organizational Psychology, 88*(2), 1–22. doi:10.1111/joop.12128

Wrzesniewski, A., and Dutton, J. E. (2001). Crafting a job: Revisioning employees as active crafters of their work. *The Academy of Management Review, 26*(2), 179–201. doi:10.2307/259118

Chapter 9

Arts-Based Wellness

Creative Strategies for Care

Jackie Gagné

Jackie Gagné is a vice principal in the St James-Assiniboia School Division in Winnipeg. She is an enthusiastic supporter of arts programming in public schools and believes that all children should be immersed in engaging arts-based experiences through-out their education. Jackie is a former arts and inte-grated arts coordinator for the division. She enjoys time with family, playing piano and guitar, painting, listening to music, live events, and long drives in the countryside.

> The aim of art is to represent not the outward appearance
> of things, but their inward significance.
> —*Aristotle*

The arts have a fascinating ability to elicit certain responses in our brains. If you have ever attended a concert with thousands of other people who share the same musical tastes, you know what it feels like when those endorphins are released as your favourite tune is being played. The sense of community and pure joy of being in the thick of the crowd, singing loud and proud, swaying your body, and shining your phone's flashlight. Those feel-good chemicals in the brain are travelling freely, producing positive psychological effects. Experiences such as these can put the rock in your rock 'n' roll!

The meanings attached to arts experiences are as unique as the individuals taking it all in. Music may be strategically chosen to stir up positive emotional responses deep within the listener, from the rush of exciting music when your favourite team scores a goal to the calm of background tunes in restaurants, but it will evoke something different in each of us.

In this chapter, the benefits of engaging in arts-based experiences for both teachers and students are considered, because teacher wellness has an impact on student wellness. Equally, the learning activities that teachers do with a focus on student well-being also have the power to enhance the teachers' well-being. They are interconnected.

In this chapter, you will be encouraged to see yourself as an artist in a variety of forms that you may not have considered until now. We will also look at specific examples of how fostering well-being in arts classrooms has brought about teacher and student wellness. Whether you are an arts teacher or a classroom teacher, I hope you will be inspired to nourish your soul and the souls of your students by bringing arts experiences into your daily life and learning spaces.

 For me, my traditional and ceremonial work is a positive and spiritual journey. I may get a bear gifted to me or someone contacts me about a deceased bear, but it could also be any animal. They ask me to take care of it, and so this means honouring the physical being and spirit of the bear. I will offer tobacco, prayer, and song, depending on my own feelings at the time. I come in contact with the spirit of the animal. I ask for permission and guidance from Creator and the spirits to use the parts of the animal, whether it be the fur, the fat to make bear grease for medicine and healing, the claws, the skull, or the bones and ribs for drum handles and tools. For me, these are all healing and honouring activities that ground me and help me to feel well.—*Elder Kipling*

This Is Your Brain on Arts

The arts have a way of evoking an intuitive response from deep within the self. Many have experienced listening to a piece of music that transcends time and conjures up particular responses. Human beings engage in the arts in ways that are uniquely interpretive and emotive. At times, memories elicit feelings of love, joy, energy, or laughter. At other times, emotions such as sorrow, fear, or anger can be triggered (Elliot and Silverman, 2015). As such, art, "whether in the form of painting, dance, music or other outlets, offers another way to process vulnerable emotions and, as a result, builds resilience" (Schwartz, 2016, p. 156).

I often find myself sitting at my piano or strumming my guitar, playing music that stirs my emotions. Certain artists evoke memories. Songs by the Guess Who and by Neil Young take me back to my childhood, to the farm in Southern Manitoba where my uncles and I would build forts, feed the animals, ride horses, and play on the back 40 in derelict vehicles. Those fond memories of my grandparents and family, brought forth through my own hands, release feel-good chemicals that bring me joy. They positively affect my well-being.

My mother's death in 2010 was the single most traumatic event I have ever experienced. My sisters and I planned a Celebration of Life, inviting family and friends to join us as we honoured the woman who left an enduring imprint on our souls. We decided that I would play piano and we daughters would sing "Let It Be," inviting the participants to sing along with us. It was a way for all of us to break bread with family and friends, bringing us all closer together. This one act of singing together, sharing our collective sorrow at this loss, helped to begin the healing process. Our wellness journey had begun.

I remember the feeling when Paul McCartney began playing the opening notes of "Let It Be" during his concert tour in Winnipeg in 2018. My endorphins went wild. It was as if a choir of thousands had suddenly burst into song. That is your brain on arts. All those lovely neurotransmitters are making connections and sending messages that everything is going to be all right, and there will be an answer. And when you are engaged in the act of singing, it "calms the heart and boosts endorphin levels" (Blumberg, 2018, quoting Daniel H. Pink). Singing together and attending live arts events adjust my mental well-being and connect my inner soul to another time and place.

Neuroesthetics is a relatively new area of scientific study focused on the neurobiological basis of the arts. It uses "brain imaging, brain wave technology, and biofeedback to gather scientific evidence of how we respond to the arts" (Martin, 2020, p. 3). This innovative research, conceived by neuroscientist Semir Zeki in the 1990s, suggests that when we are immersed in arts experiences, there is a fantastical light show in the brain when the pleasure chemicals dopamine, serotonin, and oxytocin are released. Engaging ourselves and our students in the visual arts, drama, dance, and music are fundamental to our mental and emotional health.

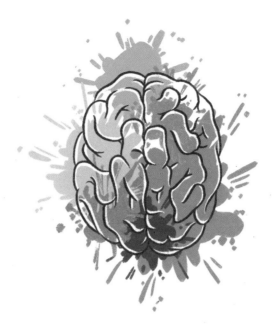

The act of hands-on art-making is as important to your health as nutrition, exercise, and meditation (Malchiodi, 2015). Actively making art has been shown to increase positive thoughts and feelings, decrease depression, and reduce stress responses in the brain. Educators can heal and maintain well-being through creative means as part of your daily routines, both in your personal lives and in classrooms. Think about yourself as a child, colouring and making sure you stayed in the lines. It was a calming activity that could keep you focused and your mental health in balance.

In a study about the effects of art on mental and physical well-being, MRIs were examined to understand the effect on the brain at a neural level (Bolwerk et al., 2014). One group of participants were art evaluators and the other half were engaged in art production. The results demonstrated that the production group showed greater spatial improvement in functional connectivity to the frontal and parietal cortices—areas of the brain related to psychological resilience. In other words, making art improves mental resilience. The power of the arts to help control stress is remarkable. Imagine yourself engaged in the act of producing art. Maybe it is colouring or sketching. Whatever activity you choose to do, notice how your brain and body calm. In this moment, give yourself permission to create.

Reflect and Respond

Brainstorm all the ways you can "keep the rock in your rock 'n' roll" through an arts experience. Mindfully explore your relationship to art.

- What art form inspires you? Maybe it is painting or listening to a piece of music that makes you want to dance. Maybe it's designing floor plans or arranging flowers.
- Try it now. Take note of how you feel when you explore and create. This is your brain on arts!
- In what other ways can you express yourself artistically and create a fantastical light show in your brain? Are you ready to try something new?

Wellness Challenges

Educators experience many challenges in their daily lives. There are times when my colleagues share their personal experiences and there are times when they put on a happy face after a traumatic event. One never truly knows how others are feeling or what may have taken place before they arrive at school. Similarly, the students in our classrooms are entering the school with experiences and situations that challenge their mental wellness.

The well-being of our staff and students is in a constant state of flux. Personal loss and trauma come in many forms—death, divorce, and more recently, the challenges associated with a pandemic. Many suffer combinations of significant loss that intensify the weight on their hearts and souls. Each person is unique and deals with stress and wellness differently.

The good news is that the arts are a welcoming space where engaging in wellness strategies for both staff and students is possible and encouraged. For those colleagues who shared their stories with me, the common thread of their journeys to wellness was that there was an arts community to support them when they were suffering. Moreover, there was an arts community to inspire them as they went about their daily lives. This approach of being proactive about wellness through an arts-based focus is supported by research:

Studies on the connection between art, healing, and health show that artistic self-expression reduces stress and anxiety and increases in positive emotions. Other studies show an improved focus on positive life experiences, self-worth, and social identity. Arts activities also play a role in developing resilience and mental wellbeing. (Naiman, 2021)

Current experts on burnout suggest that creative expressions are a tool that can help us pass through the stress cycle to the "rest and digest" state (Nagoski and Nagoski, 2020). This research affirms the value of integrating the arts into workplace wellness programs and initiatives to provide one more approach to positive well-being for school staff.

Fostering Wellness through Dance

Dance is the hidden language of the soul.
—*Martha Graham*

The dance teacher knew that the exercise would require sensitivity and care, as his students could be rattled, maybe even triggered. He had prepared them by sharing his journey of being labelled and bullied in high school, in a time and place when diversity and inclusion were not considered basic human rights by much of society. In the early 1990s, the school community had yet to evolve in respecting and accepting all individuals regardless of gender and sexual orientation.

Relationships built on trust, safety, and belonging had been firmly established with this teacher's group of students as he had taught many of them for several years. His goal was to instill resiliency and encourage students to "burn down the field beforehand so they could grow something beautiful." The exercise they were beginning would prove a uniquely individual experience. Yet teacher and students would find that, working together, their well-being grew into something beautiful.

The dance studio was quiet as students studied themselves in the mirror that stretched from one end of the room to the other. They represented a cross-section of humanity, of various sizes, shapes, and skills. Once they had the chance to get that picture of themselves in their heads, they traced their body shapes onto the full-length studio mirrors using chalk markers. As the students stood back and looked at the outlines of their bodies, the teacher asked them to use words to describe themselves. He asked them to recall words that people had called them, words that labelled them, and words to describe the way they thought they were perceived. As they printed outside the chalk lines, words like "fat," "ugly," "stupid," and "crybaby" were revealed. (Because this activity had the potential to trigger emotions related to self-esteem, body image, trauma, or grief, the teacher made sure that students knew they had access to a school counsellor.)

Next, he asked them to look inside the chalk lines to think about who they thought they were. He asked them to write words that described their positive strengths, the parts of their personalities and lives that the outside world might not see but that they knew were examples of how incredible they were. Words such as "comedian," "intelligent," and "respectful" were revealed. Students then reflected on the words outside and within their chalk outlines. This allowed them to see that the words that people use to label us are not truly reflective of who we are.

What the teacher had given himself and his students that day was more than perfecting the pirouette. He had provided an experience of deep connection with the group as a whole. Together, through the lesson, they identified the "fields that needed to be burned" before healing could take place. They were a community of individuals who had experienced labels and loss of self through the perceptions of others. Thus began a process of healing inner spirits and emotional scars caused by words. As he guided his students in reflection, self-discovery, and creating connections, he was on a journey of his own, mending his wounds. It was a process of healing and learning resiliency for everyone, all through dance.

After months of introspection, carefully thought-out lessons, and dance rehearsals, the class production of "This Is Me," from *The Greatest Showman,* hit the stage. The onlookers experienced the shedding of layers of costumes until all that was left was the students in their nude-coloured bodysuits with the injurious words printed in bold, black marker. The emotional performance precipitated tears from the performers and observers. All were touched by what they had just participated in. It was a genuine human experience, spoken through the art of dance.

The experience provided a forum for members of the class to come to terms with negative perceptions and feelings of self that, once revealed, paved the way to wellness through an understanding of resiliency. This example of a teacher's wellness journey, in conjunction with his students' wellness journey, demonstrates the need for human connectedness while healing trauma. As teachers consider how to address their challenges and deeply rooted injuries, they can support students to do the same in a safe and trusting environment.

Reflect and Respond

In the "This Is Me" activity, the teacher and students recorded harsh things that people had said to them or that they had said to themselves. However, these students also knew things to be true about themselves that were affirming.

- Consider the words you have heard used to describe you, and the words you have used to describe yourself.
- Sketch a body outline.
- Inside the body outline, record positive statements based on affirming words, for example: "I am a good friend." "I love to laugh out loud." "I am working on being more kind to myself."

Fostering Wellness through Visual Arts

> I saw the angel in the marble and carved until I set him free.
> —*Michelangelo*

The art teacher's world was spinning out of control. Stress, anxiety, and burnout dominated her daily experiences. These were compounded by grief associated with the death of her beloved sister and her impending divorce. But she found some solace in her carefully designed art room. A special place for her and her students, it was filled, floor to ceiling, with hundreds of colourful creations, works in progress, and completed pieces. It was a room that inspired and allowed students to unleash their creativity.

From her sacred space, she gathered several framed canvases and tubes of paint and set out for home to begin her journey of healing. She decided to begin her wellness journey by painting a portrait of herself, using colour to express how she was feeling at the time. For months, she continued painting portraits of herself and posting them online. Alert social media followers could see that minute details were changed with each new portrait. Her eyeglass frames were light, then dark. Tattoo art was added to her features. She titled one of her portraits "Bruised." Colours changed. First white. Then yellow, blue, and finally green. The process of healing was not tied up with a tidy bow, moving from anger to wellness, or from dark to light. The portraits reflected her fluctuations in mental wellness, showing the natural process of healing, with all its setbacks and forward movement.

She started thinking about how her journey to wellness through art therapy could be a starting point to help her students practise art skills in the context of wellness and mindfulness. Thus, the Art Exploration course was born. She chose the theme of "The Others," encouraging students to sketch, record, and brainstorm who the "others" were in their lives and why they mattered. She asked them to explore, through art, how they could heal negative perceptions of themselves, as well as the effects of others' perceptions of them. Students were able to choose their art media; they could draw, paint, collage, use clay, or whatever worked for them. They were encouraged to use the media as a way of experimenting with their feelings and giving their piece a voice.

At every point in this self-directed learning course, the teacher conducted wellness checks with students as they expressed their thoughts and feelings. She got the school guidance counsellor involved so that students had access to a resource for coping strategies if needed.

The students were able to express themselves in ways that the teacher could not have predicted. Art was not about creating the same product or following the same process for each student. It provided a creative means through which students could set free the "angel in the marble" at a personal level. For the teacher, engaging in the self-portrait activity helped her express her emotions through colour. She found that every brushstroke was therapeutic. It provided a creative outlet that fostered her journey toward healing and mental well-being.

Reflect and Respond
- Think about a time when your wellness was challenged. What would your self-portrait have looked like? Visualize or draw it. Add colour.
- Think about another time when you experienced a positive sense of well-being. What would your self-portrait have looked like? Visualize or draw it. Add colour.

If you find drawing faces challenging, as I do, think of using shapes to help guide you in your drawing.

Fostering Wellness through Early Years Music

Music is the electrical soil in which the spirit lives, thinks and invents.
—Beethoven

The early years music teacher remembers being a complete mess after her loss. It was the end of her relationship and the end of a life experience abroad. She decided to move back to Manitoba and take time to get her life sorted out. One of the first things she turned to as a healing outlet was music. She got involved in a church choir and played in a band, enjoying the feeling of camaraderie as they made music together and for others. She listened to music on a live-stream everywhere she went to calm and focus her thoughts.

She ended up picking up the guitar and piano again, as she found much joy and expression in playing and singing. She also wrote several original songs, weaving poetry and melody together, and found it very therapeutic. One day, while substitute teaching, she taught *The Little Red Hen* story with an accompanying Orff arrangement (an approach that combines music, speech, movement, and drama). It filled her heart with joy to see the excitement on the students' faces as they wove storytelling and music into a magical journey. She just knew this was the perfect time to become an early years music specialist.

She faced challenges in building an inner-city music program and working with at-risk children. She incorporated dance, visual arts, and drama into her music class. Many classes were spent listening to a piece of music, eyes closed, soaking in the sounds. Then they would draw and dream and use their imaginations as they listened to the music again. They shared ideas about what the composer might be thinking or feeling, and about how they were thinking and feeling when listening to the piece. They used books and art visuals to explore the feelings and colours of music. Instrumental arrangements were created with opportunities for improvisation and dance.

Soon students were beginning to participate more, collaborating on ideas for creating music, and were better able to practise self-regulation. Music class was creating positive pathways in the brains and bodies of her students—and herself. Students were thinking critically and creatively while collaborating with their peers. Music class had become, for both the teacher and her students, a place of solace, peace, belonging, and wellness.

For many Indigenous Peoples, the drum represents the heartbeat of Mother Earth, but also the beating heart of our mother when we are in the womb. In my community, we are told by the old people that if we ever want to soothe a baby, we play a drum and try to find a beat in the drum that brings back memories of their time in the womb.—*Elder Kipling*

Fostering Wellness through the Dramatic Arts

The drama teacher says that musical theatre is her special place. When not attending to a loved one who has significant health-care needs, it is her home away from home where she finds shelter and a supportive community. The stage is a place where she and her students can identify with a character, build confidence to communicate and share stories, and have fun through music and dance. It is a place where reason, respect, and responsibility come together, sometimes after conflict. She feels the benefits to both her own and her students' mental wellness. The stage helps develop leadership skills needed for children to grow into flourishing, contributing members of society through creative problem-solving. It also fosters wellness and builds community among its members when they are not on stage.

As a director and teacher, she arrives an hour before call time and remains long after the rehearsal is over. She is there to direct, yes, but also to be human, to be social, and to check in to find out how her community is doing emotionally. She listens, exchanges stories, and engages in authentic conversation, gradually building a culture of safety and belonging. In this way, everyone knows who to push for more emotion during the scene and who to afford more space. The ideal is a healthy community that sustains wellness and supports students and the director alike on and off the stage and in challenging times.

The director sees the entire process leading up to the production as a journey toward wellness, for both the teacher and for students. Making and maintaining connections with all members of the drama family—the cast, musicians, dancers, stage managers, sound production crew, and technicians—is key to fostering personal wellness. Those connections forge a sense of belonging for participants and have a positive effect on the emotional and psychological needs of the group. It's a reciprocal interchange, where mental wellness is sustained by relationships and the feelings of safety and belonging that are experienced in theatre.

Reflect and Respond

- Think about your personal and professional life. In which part(s) of your life do you feel a culture of safety and belonging?
- How does this help to sustain and support your wellness?

Wellness in My Music Classroom

In my classroom, I often focused on wellness using the auditory and visual senses as stimuli for mindful reflection with my students. This form of guided imagery was especially effective as a way of helping them to breathe and relax their bodies. For example, I would play a piece of music, such as Beethoven's *Romance for violin and orchestra No. 2 in F major, Op. 50,* or I would display a piece of art by Monet that depicts a calm scene with nature. I used these, both works that I had experienced personally as having calming effects, to set the tone for introspection.

Other times, I would ask my students to close their eyes and listen as I used a soft, calming voice that allowed them to mindfully engage with their imaginations. Here is an example:

> Close your eyes. Take a deep breath through your nose, now exhale through your mouth. Breathe in through your nose again, then out through your mouth. One more time. Now think of a place that is peaceful. There are tall trees full of leaves. You can hear the gentle tinkle of water. You follow the sound through the tall grass. There are colourful wildflowers surrounding you. You are very relaxed and feeling happy. You can see water in the distance. It looks as shiny as glass. You sit down in the grass and watch the water flow. You are thinking of things that bring you joy and make you smile. Stay in that place awhile.

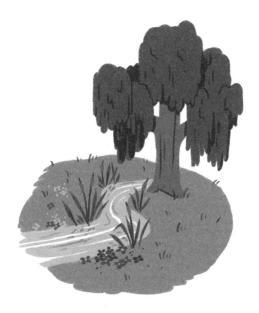

Guided imagery is good for establishing an atmosphere that supports self-regulation in the learning environment (Shardlow, 2015). Using this strategy in my classroom helped my students regulate their emotions so that they could feel calm and comfortable in their bodies.

This technique is a strategy for mindfulness that I use for myself as well. It helps to calm my mind and body before sleep or when I am facing a mental well-being challenge and need to catch a breath.

 | The Earth, nature, always inspires and heals.—*Elder Kipling*

Beginning Your Arts Journey

I have had the most insightful experiences working with classroom teachers, arts specialists, and artists in schools. These folks continuously have a profound impact, transforming learning and developing people in their classrooms, on stages, and in studios. They share a common belief that engaging our students in arts experiences in all curricular areas can deepen learning and understanding of the world around us. They feel the magical healing effects when they are actively participating in art experiences and share that well-being with their students.

If you have little or no experience in the arts or with arts integration, I encourage you to begin the process of seeing yourself through a different lens, as an artist. We are all creative in different ways. Some maintain a beautifully landscaped yard. Others have inventively designed a man cave, equipped with vintage signage and lights. Some can cook up a fabulous meal and serve it in an aesthetically pleasing way. These are all examples that demonstrate creativity and imagination. I invite you to begin to think of yourself as an artist.

Reflect and Respond

Wherever you are in your arts journey, I invite you to reflect on a form of play you engaged in during your childhood. You may have enjoyed playing an instrument, doodling, or painting.

- Reflect on something you've created or designed that brings out the artist in you.
- Consider revisiting the activity that brought you joy. The idea is to allow yourself time to play and to focus on the actual process of engaging in an art activity.

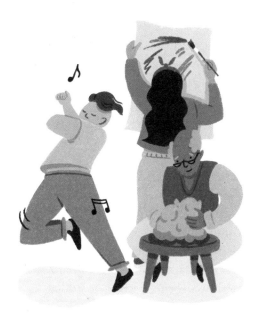

Consider introducing an art element into your teaching where you and your students are actively participating. For example, dance could be a way to discover planetary motion. Consider sculpture to talk about mass and space. These cross-curricular connections could add a spark of excitement and curiosity for you and your students. The possibilities are endless. Take note of how you and your students connect and respond through art experiences and how mental wellness is fostered. Notice also how it affects your own experience of teaching.

The arts have a magical way of making connections in the brain that can heal us and help to maintain wellness. The arts build relationships and a sense of belonging, which are fundamental to fostering well-being. These benefits are crucial to developing a world of kind and caring individuals who can collaborate to make their communities and the world a better place.

Closing Thoughts

I am grateful to my colleagues who have shared not only their strategies and lessons for fostering the well-being of their students but also how embracing the arts has brought about a healing process when their mental wellness was being challenged. Permission to play and explore through creativity offers another way to process emotional responses and can assist in healing past trauma. Bringing arts to your personal lives and classrooms as part of your daily routines will increase wellness while reducing stress. It is not enough to simply evaluate art as a consumer. Actively making art improves mental resilience, releases those feel-good chemicals, and is important nutrition for your well-being. I wish you all a wonderful journey in all your artistic endeavours! Teacher, be well!

Reflect and Respond
As you embark on your journey of wellness through the arts, I invite you to:
- Use guided imagery as a tool for reflection.
- Allow yourself and your students time to "play" in a specific arts area.
- Experiment with a variety of art media to express your emotions.
- Conduct routine check-ins with yourself, your students, and your colleagues.

References and Further Reading

Blumberg, Y. (2018, February 23). *Singing in a choir could be "the new exercise"—Here's the surprising science behind why.* CNBC make it. https://www.cnbc.com/2018/02/23/daniel-h-pink-shares-why-choral-singing-benefits-health-like-exercise.html

Bolwerk, A., Mack-Andrick, J., Lang, F. R., Dörfler, A., & Maihöfner, C. (2014, December 22). How art changes your brain: Differential effects of visual art production and cognitive art evaluation on functional brain connectivity. *PLOS ONE, 9*(7), e1001035. https://doi.org/10.1371/journal.pone.0101035

Elliott, D., & Silverman, M. (2015). *Music matters: A philosophy of music education* (2nd ed.). Oxford University Press.

Malchiodi, C. (2015, December 31). Creativity as a wellness practice. *Psychology Today.* https://www.psychologytoday.com/ca/blog/arts-and-health/201512/creativity-wellness-practice

Martin, B. H. (2020, June 9). Brain research shows the arts promote mental health. *The Conversation.* https://theconversation.com/brain-research-shows-the-arts-promote-mental-health-136668

Nagoski, E., & Nagoski, A. (2020). *Burnout: The secret to unlocking the stress cycle.* Ballantine Books.

Naiman, L. (2021, January 3). *Enhance mental health and workplace wellness with art and creativity.* Creativity at work. https://www.creativityatwork.com/what-is-the-connection-between-creativity-and-workplace-wellness/

Schwartz, A. (2016). *The complex PTSD workbook.* Althea Press.

Seligman, M. E. P. (2013). *Flourish: A visionary new understanding of happiness and well-being.* Atria.

Shardlow, G. (2015, November 18). Integrating mindfulness in your classroom curriculum. *Edutopia.* https://www.edutopia.org/blog/integrating-mindfulness-in-classroom-curriculum-giselle-shardlow

Chapter 10

Bringing Our Voices Together
Classroom Relationships for Wellness

Monika Rosney and Richelle North Star Scott

Monika Cichosz Rosney, BA, BEd, is a Polish-born settler with more than a decade of experience teaching students of all ages, from infants to adults. Navigating multiple cultures from childhood and learning about her privilege, place, intergenerational stories, and resilience informs Monika's wellness journey. Teaching relationships shaped Monika's change of focus from academics to healing and social justice. Now, working on her Master of Marriage and Family Therapy, she supports culturally congruent community care as a powerful foundation for self-care, equity, and wellness. Monika is grateful for continued spiritual development as a relational therapist, new parent, and contributing author. She lives in Winnipeg on Treaty 1 territory with her spouse and child.

Knowledge Keeper and writer **Richelle North Star Scott** (Giiwedinong Anong) is of Anishinaabe and Métis descent, and her Ancestors are from St Peter's Reserve. See more on page 10.

The authors of this chapter, Monika and North Star, share their thoughts about classroom wellness. Their conversation appears here as a dialogue. Monika also interviewed a third person, Mojgan, and shares her story as well.

Bringing Voices Together

Monika: This chapter includes the voices of three teachers with unique experiences and understandings of wellness. I have been honoured to build relationships and collaborate with the two other contributors to this chapter. Over the years, Knowledge Keeper North Star has generously shared a wealth of teachings with my classes. I met Mojgan when we worked together while teaching English to adult Newcomers who arrived as immigrants and refugees. We have woven our stories together to provide diverse perspectives on teacher wellness.

In each of our wellness journeys as teachers, we have experienced the healing power of relationships with students, colleagues, and the land. This chapter is about how these relationships, supported by class wellness practices, can support teacher well-being and workplace wellness. We share how we infuse wellness practices into our teaching. These practices support student and teacher wellness by building deeper relationships with ourselves, each other, and the land. Our work as teachers fills us up when students have a voice and choice, and feel deeply seen and heard.

Monika's Perspective on Wellness

Monika: More than a decade ago, I attended a wellness workshop as a teacher candidate. After hearing statistics about teacher burnout, I left thinking, "Why are so many teachers leaving the profession in the first five years?" Since that day, as I struggled to balance and be well, I experienced many wellness wake-up calls.

One such call was early in my career when I worked too late at school. As I entered the dark hallway for supplies, I was lit by the bright beam of a flashlight. I had unknowingly set off the silent alarm, and two police officers had arrived. One checked my identification while the other asked when I had started work that day. They walked me out, then watched me brush the snow off my car and drive away. Maybe it's against the law to work that late. Lesson learned.

My path to wellness, like so much of life, has not been linear. To become more myself, I reflect on trauma, culture, and healing. It is an ongoing process. Recently, I experienced my most powerful wellness wake-up call: change. I became a parent and a therapist amid the pandemic. At the same time, I experienced distance in relationships with people while reconnecting to the land. With these changes, I needed more than ever to remember the wellness lessons I had previously learned in relationships with students and colleagues. Wellness requires multiple systems including, for me, a supportive school culture and my personal work. Class wellness practices also support both student and teacher wellness (Garcia, n.d.). As we teach the next seven generations, we teachers can support our well-being by learning from our students and colleagues and benefiting from these caring relationships.

North Star's Perspective on Wellness

North Star: As an Indigenous teacher, I believe that when we teach from the heart and the spirit, we are not only taking care of the students in our classroom, but we are also taking care of ourselves. Relationships built on a foundation of trust are places where students have an authentic voice and participate in deep listening. We all need good, positive relationships with our colleagues, students, and ourselves.

Having a positive relationship with yourself means having a deep relationship with the Earth. It takes all kinds of relationships to keep our mental health in check. That is what is meant by balance. Indigenous Peoples all across Turtle Island have had committed relationships with the land, water, and animals that live in their territories. My relationship with the Earth supports me in my relationship with myself, other teachers, and my students.

I also need to mention that Indigenous Peoples love to laugh. So, part of being honest with my students is to tell them funny stories about my life or something ridiculous that has happened to me out on the land.

With this framework, I have come to understand that true healing comes from a place of deep knowing and deep listening. This is a vision we want for all beings on the Earth—to be well beings.

Mojgan's Story of Work and Wellness

Monika: I first met Mojgan when we worked together at Peaceful Village. She now works as an English as an Additional Language (EAL) teacher and case manager at a public high school with Newcomer families and international students.

In 2005, Mojgan immigrated to Winnipeg from Iran with her spouse and two daughters. Mojgan's degrees from Iran were not accepted. She and her spouse were required to study in Winnipeg to obtain "Canadian education and experience," which she experienced as a form of cultural assimilation (personal communication). While completing two full-time years of study for her Bachelor of Education, Mojgan worked three jobs: as an education assistant, as a teacher at Peaceful Village, and as a support worker for DASCH, a non-profit organization in Winnipeg. With help only from one family member, Mojgan and her family faced many challenges. They had little savings in the bank. Learning and working in multiple languages, navigating various social systems and cultures, Winnipeg weather, and guilt and worry about leaving family behind in Iran were all mentally exhausting. Their daughters faced bullying and discrimination at school and were offered minimal EAL teaching support.

Mojgan described "a very unclear future. There was no light, just darkness, because you don't know what's going to happen to you and your kids, and you decided to bring them here." Over the years, she and her spouse made it through the dark times together, providing a new life with greater opportunities for their daughters. Mojgan's personal experience has fuelled her professional passion to support Newcomer students and families.

When Mojgan shared with me her story about the power of relationships and self-care, she focused on resilience, balance, and team support. This approach helps her in one of the great juggling acts of a teacher: supporting students from different backgrounds. With her international students, she found her assumptions about family wealth and ease challenged as she learned about family separation, parental isolation, and the tremendous family pressure on students to achieve top grades. The refugee families Mojgan works with experience Newcomer obstacles as well, but they are also overcoming trauma, safety issues, and sudden loss of community.

There is much pressure on Mojgan to teach these students academics, even when what they need most are healing and layers of support. She responds to their trauma stories as well as their need for learning. She also educates colleagues on trauma-informed practices.

Amid these challenges, Mojgan recognizes the role her wellness plays. "I need to take care of my wellness because I want to help more kids. I want to be a person they can trust and talk to, who might understand them better. If I break, I can't help, and people keep coming. I need to take care of myself."

By seeking her students' strengths, Mojgan is reminded of her strength. Her focus on resilience allows her to experience empathy and gratitude. She recognizes the pressure her international students are under from their families to achieve top grades and this brings greater appreciation for the sources of support in her life. By recognizing students' courage in seeking help when they are struggling with family demands, Mojgan is reminded of how far she has come in her journey to provide opportunities for her family. When working with refugee families, Mojgan responds with empathy and understanding as she prays for students' missing or waiting family members, while also honouring their efforts to make a life for themselves.

She recalls a widowed mother of seven, studying English, who is so happy and proud to greet Mojgan in school. When Mojgan misses her daughters, who are now grown and live far away, she thinks of this family. She is grateful for the sacrifices she and her spouse made so their daughters would have greater safety and security.

When it comes to the pressure on her to teach academics, Mojgan focuses on students' achievements. For example, the joy students experience when they can finally write "I am from Iraq" inspires Mojgan's gratitude. Bearing witness to their accomplishments empowers her. She replenishes herself by focusing on what builds her students' resilience. Their small gains, strengths, contributions, and employable skills that will allow them to support their families bring rewards for her as well.

Working with refugee families and international students requires balance. Mojgan limits her exposure to news and books about crime, violence, and war. Too much exposure to such media can make sympathy for her refugee students her primary focus, which may prevent them from moving forward. At home, Mojgan connects with her family by talking to her daughters and her mother on weekly video chats. She focuses on joy and slowing down through exercise, yoga, and mindful colouring books. Mojgan also finds balance during the school day through the team support she shares with her colleagues. With one colleague, she gets physically active during the lunch hour on exercise machines and outdoor river walks.

Team support is important, especially when facing challenges with colleagues. Mojgan often acts as a servant-leader, educating colleagues on trauma-informed teaching practices—sometimes unexpectedly. For example, Mojgan heard assumptions from school staff that an absent student was lazy. Meanwhile, this student was caring for their surviving siblings as the family grieved the death anniversary of their murdered children. It can be difficult to respond to stories of trauma while also educating colleagues about what conversations, symbols, and assumptions can re-traumatize students. Yet Mojgan has the support and understanding of her administrators. She also appreciates the two counsellors who support her own and students' wellness by teaching calming grounding techniques. Support also comes from Mojgan's teaching team of three; they bring each other coffee, consult about students, and problem-solve together. The team provides each other with emotional support and, most importantly, they know they are not alone.

North Star: We can design elaborate lesson plans, but current events, such as the discovery of 215 children's graves at the Kamloops Residential School, can set us off on another course. When an Ontario resident used a car as a weapon to purposefully run over a Muslim family, killing four of the five members, that tragedy sparked intense conversations in our classrooms. When we are working with Indigenous and Newcomer students, these kinds of discoveries may bring up old wounds. This can create opportunities to talk truthfully about the traumas that have surfaced because of where we all come from and where we currently live. We can help both Indigenous and Newcomer children make powerful connections with each other.

Talking Circles

North Star: We in teaching know that we need to support each other in difficult times. There are many paths to wellness, and when we choose relational paths, we experience the benefits of community support and intention. We motivate each other to care for our wellness, acknowledge when we are struggling, and know we are not alone. The Elders tell us, "My child, you need to remember how to listen." When we all practise the art of listening, we can feel deeply seen and heard at any age. Talking Circles help us to put the art of listening into action.

The Indigenous protocols of a Talking Circle are passed down from Elders and Knowledge Keepers. These practices can be adopted for classroom use. Please seek out an Elder or Knowledge Keeper to guide you, as these protocols have been gifted to them from the land. If you do not know the protocols for Elders in your territory, ask for guidance.

Another thing to consider when using a Talking Circle in your wellness program is the Indigenous idea of consent. In Anishinaabe culture, we never demand that our community members participate. This becomes scary for some teachers because it is about letting go of control. We all have students in our classrooms who might not consent to what we teach. Often these are the students who wander the hallways. This teaching of consent is a reminder that we have sovereignty over our bodies, which is essential for safety.

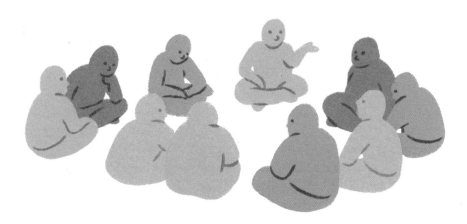

Monika: The Talking Circle is the most powerful relational practice I've experienced that supports wellness at any grade level. In a Talking Circle, we sit facing each other, often outside on the land. We pass around a Grandparent rock, which is a stone or rock that is used to focus attention, a Talking stick, or a feather. These are gifts from the land. The person who holds the Grandparent rock is the only person speaking and no one is to interrupt. As each person receives the object, they speak for as long as they wish and then pass the rock to the next person once they have finished. If someone does not want to share, they can choose not to consent and instead pass the rock to the next person. The people in the circle can decide what to talk about and when the circle is over. The rock might be passed around multiple times until everyone is finished speaking, or until an issue is resolved.

Because of the time constraints of the school day—a colonial structure—we sometimes finish a Talking Circle on another day. We show respect by listening and responding without judgment. We speak honestly and truthfully, showing support with our body language and facial expressions, and keeping what is said in the circle private. The Talking Circle encourages participants to formulate thoughts before voicing ideas, speak from the heart with confidence and clarity, and practise patience, compassion, and curiosity when actively listening. In these ways, it develops strength of character (Katz and Lamoureux, 2018).

In my experience, the Talking Circle allowed us to practise the teaching of Respect and to learn more about each other. My class and I had Talking Circles weekly and many students looked forward to this time. Sometimes students would call a Talking Circle to resolve an issue as a class community. At times, listening was uncomfortable, and interruptions happened as we learned. This practice requires a time investment. That commitment helped me since I often spoke as a teacher and felt pressure to follow a schedule. Listening without interrupting or judging allows us to develop our empathy and curiosity, and it is especially challenging when we are accustomed to interactions of efficiency.

North Star: I was once given a fantastic teaching by Elder Myra Laramee. She said that if you ask someone how they are doing, you had better be prepared to stop and listen. How often do we greet our colleagues after winter break by saying, "Hello, how are you?" and then hurrying past them to get to our next task, not really listening to their reply? They may even shout out a quick "I'm fine" (even if they are not okay) as they make a beeline for the next item on their to-do list. These "efficient" interactions have unfortunately taught us to not listen to each other.

The land reminds us how to listen. When I am out on the land, whether just to breathe fresh air, reintroduce myself to my natural relatives, or out harvesting medicines, I need to be safe. I need to listen for the animals whose territory I am wandering in. If I am harvesting on the land, I need to announce my arrival and intent to the land. Once introductions are done, I always ask, "Is it okay to harvest sage here today?"

I teach my students that sometimes the land says no! But students always ask, how do you listen to the land?

I tell them that I believe we have always had the ability to listen to the land, water, and animals. We used to speak their language, but we have forgotten how to listen. I tell them to think about the stories the European Ancestors called fairy tales. In these stories, the animals spoke, and we understood what they were saying. In Indigenous storytelling, animals not only spoke to each other, but they also spoke to us, and we understood them. Inside this teaching is a lesson about listening and remembering.

Unfortunately, many of us have removed ourselves from our natural state of being, which is to listen and respond to nature. By using Talking Circles, the focus can once again be on listening, and we can learn to listen with authenticity and understanding.

Monika: Talking Circles helped us slow down to the natural rhythms of the land and to recognize each other's wholeness. My students saw me as a human being with a life outside of school. Sometimes we learned about others' quiet joys and heart-wrenching struggles that we might otherwise have missed. This knowledge helped us to celebrate each other's strengths and to respond with empathy more often during challenging times.

Reflect and Respond
- Do you feel deeply heard? When you don't feel listened to, what do you do to feel heard?
- Go outside somewhere alone and ground yourself to the Earth. Once you feel grounded, use your voice in a way that carries it from your feet up to your throat. Sound your voice! At first, your voice may be soft, but then, when you feel comfortable, slowly sound your voice loudly, as if to the moon.

Mindfulness: Listening in Another Way

Monika: When I first started mindfulness practice, I found it uncomfortable. Slowing down brought up painful and uncomfortable emotions that I had numbed with work and staying busy. Mindfulness brought the beginning of wisdom to care for myself in a new way. Emotions that arise need to be supported with compassion. With my students, I assumed laughing, commenting, zoning out, or falling asleep were signs that we were not good at mindfulness practice or that it wasn't working for us.

For my students and myself, I learned to let go of striving for perfection. I tried to embrace the purpose of mindfulness practice: the imperfect process of gently, repeatedly returning our attention to ourselves, in the same way as we listen to someone speak in the Talking Circle. Practising mindfulness on the land can help us connect to natural rhythms. It can enhance our ability to attend to the process of being present, rather than focusing on an outcome. Think about what you read in chapter 3, "Making Sense of Mindfulness." All these practices benefit both students and teachers when implemented in the class setting.

North Star: As an Indigenous Kookoo (grandmother), I am aware of my mindfulness, and I'm constantly in prayer when I am out on the land. By sharing my teachings with students, I have learned to have gratitude in the most difficult of situations. I try to demonstrate how I slow down to deal with a problem and model how to be grateful for the things we take for granted. I hope this helps students see how they can deal with conflict while remaining in a place of peace on the land. For me, mindfulness, gratitude, and relationships are partners in wellness.

Monika: One of the most powerful benefits of mindfulness for me is when I worry about a student or family after I have already done what I can do to support them. I need to do something with that energy, so I breathe deeply and send hope, love, and strength to them. In this way, I offer trust in others' sovereignty over their own lives and focus on living my life. Mindfulness practice can also reduce reactivity, increase concentration, and strengthen willpower (McGonigal, 2012).

Most valuable for relationships, we learn to listen with curiosity as we calm our nervous systems (McGonigal 2012). Responding to challenging behaviours with curiosity and compassion allows our relationships to become sources of safety and healing instead of re-traumatizing (Brown, 2021). By increasing safety in our relationships, we can do the vulnerable work of living from our values, holding our boundaries, and deeply connecting with ourselves and others. This benefits our wellness (Brown 2017).

Before exploring mindfulness practices with students, I needed to learn more myself. I learned through co-teaching with student services staff, professional development, a mindfulness-based stress reduction course, and delving into research.

I began mindfulness practice by asking my students what they knew about it. We discussed benefits. We explored a variety of mindfulness practices through lessons connected to the curriculum (Katz and Lamoureux, 2018). To support our practice, we worked with a variety of focuses, such as the breath, emotions, sounds, and cultivating compassion. We were flexible in how we met our sensory needs. For example, during a seated mindfulness practice, some students moved a bit and others rocked the entire time. For some, we adjusted the length of their practice. Others engaged in mindful colouring. I learned that closing the eyes can reactivate trauma, so having the option to keep eyes open is helpful. Respecting our needs benefited everyone's wellness and supported our relationships. I was regularly reminded that supporting student wellness can have positive effects on teacher wellness and that the same practices that work for students can work for me.

We often repeated the same type of practice over a series of days or weeks. For example, when practising mindful listening, we listened to different spontaneous sounds, such as the wind, our breathing, birds, traffic, and the loudest and quietest sounds we heard. During one lesson, staff and students took turns hiding behind a divider (great for early years kids) and made different sounds, such as a pencil tapping or a drum. Students listened and guessed the sounds. I found it helpful to have a cue that mindfulness practice would begin and end, such as a singing bowl, bell, or chime. We kept the same practice structure to make it routine. When North Star would bring her drum, drumming and singing became our mindfulness practice before the lessons.

North Star: Mindfulness practices teach us to be with ourselves in stillness, to slow down and to listen in another way. To support Monika's routines of mindfulness and have a consistent structure for her students, I would always bring my drum when visiting the class for a lesson. I would often start by tapping out a consistent rhythm on the drum, a repetitive beat representing the heartbeat of Earth and healing. I would then ask the students to breathe deeply while getting their body, emotions, mind, and spirit ready for learning. Our hand drums were used by the Mothers,

Aunties, and Grandmothers to soothe and calm children after a long day. It was with these lullabies that we rocked our children to sleep and comforted them when they were out of balance with their emotions. We would hold our babies' ears near our own hearts to help them regulate their heartbeat. Drumming while hearing traditional songs being sung in Anishinaabemowin became a wellness practice in Monika's classroom.

Monika: Once we learned a variety of mindfulness practices, the class identified moments when they needed practise, such as after lunch. The idea was to make this a routine. We scheduled a few minutes of mindfulness practice to ground ourselves at this time each day. Students participated in whatever way they wanted to while respecting others' choices. Eventually, some students spontaneously practised mindfulness to help themselves regulate their emotions. They did this with me, with other students, with North Star drumming and singing (in person or on YouTube), through recorded music or voice meditation, and in creating art, song, prayer, and more. The goal was not to assimilate kids into fitting in by pretending to "feel calm," but to support and teach paths to balance and wellness that respected everyone's needs.

North Star: These kinds of classroom mindfulness practices allow students to have a choice and a voice within their classroom. This strengthens their sovereignty through consent. When we invite students to participate, we need to anticipate that they may say no. When we provide choices within a given framework, students are more likely to give their consent to what we are teaching.

Reflect and Respond
- Be mindful of the land and how you are feeling while on it. Check your Physical, Emotional, Mental, and Spiritual well-being. Touch the grasses to connect to your physical aspect. Sit down and feel your emotional self connected to the Earth. What are you thinking as your mental aspect comes into balance? Where are you spiritually? Are you feeling plugged into the energy? Are you feeling inspired? Are you feeling in awe of your surroundings? Sit in gratitude.

- Drink water and be thankful for it. Speak to it and allow it to nurture all aspects of your Sacred Hoop.
- Make time to connect to the natural rhythms of the Earth. Spend time with the stars. Find the planets in the night sky, chart the phases of the moon, or learn what time the sun comes up. Create your ceremonies around these elements to create balance and calm in your life.
- Most of all, choose you.

Lessons of Honesty

Monika: I started teaching because I loved working with kids. If you asked me what I loved, I would have said, "Their energy, their curiosity, and modelling my love of learning for them." What I love now is their whole beings—and their honesty, which has directed me to my wellness lessons. A three-year-old's frightened face taught me to forget the stern teacher's look and choose compassion. A Grade 5 student told me to go home when I looked ill. A high-school student cracked jokes to help us all relax. Many students reminded me to connect to the land by asking to learn outside. So many children have shown me how they can be unapologetically themselves and truly belong while navigating the pressure to fit in. When I worked with North Star, her way of being was a reminder of what my students have always taught me, that belonging to oneself brings belonging in relationships. And this enhances both teacher and student wellness.

North Star: I approach residential schools honestly when sharing some hard truths about broken promises and broken relationships. This led Monika's class into a conversation about residential school children and the United Nation's Rights of the Child. When teaching sensitive content, not only for the students but also for me, I remain vigilant on how I'm feeling when discussing Indigenous history. I often found that, during the lesson, as an inheritor of these dysfunctional legacies, I was triggered by the content.

Once we have a good foundation in the history of residential schools, I often tackle the idea of Reconciliation. The students in the class decided that, as part of Reconciliation, they were going to create a bulletin board on residential schools, focusing on children's rights. The bulletin board was going to be used as a teaching tool for families to spark hallway conversations.

Thanks to Monika not shying away from these difficult conversations, she often had deep and meaningful talks with her students. I was awed when an Indigenous student from her class affirmed: "I have the right to my own gender identity!" This is true inclusion if we can have conversations about groups of people that have previously been marginalized, like the LGBTTQQIASP* community. These conversations alone bring well-being to both students and educators.

Reflect and Respond
- What practices do you already participate in that help you stay grounded during difficult classroom conversations and unplanned moments?
- How can a mindfulness practice support everyone's wellness while engaging in difficult classroom conversations?
- Is there a way for you to incorporate being out on the land to help with either grounding or having difficult conversations?

Connecting to the Land

Monika: Decades ago, as a young child, I implored other kids not to break branches because it hurt trees. I was mocked for believing that trees can feel. At home, I drew trees, animals, and water with words asking for their respect and protection. As I became a mostly indoor child and teenager, I gradually internalized colonial concepts that I was separate from the land. I knew something about wellness that I forgot.

As a teacher, I often taught indoors because it was familiar and comfortable. Yet I noticed how our energy, patience, and wellness were restored when I explored teaching outdoors. I became more aware of how my actions affected the land. I started learning and taking action in my personal life and with students. We supported our wellness with composting, gardening, outdoor exercise, and dance. We learned about the land. We consumed less and used second-hand. These actions encouraged me to take further personal and political action in the face of our long-standing ecological crisis. I became more connected to the land, myself, and the human relationships that strengthened my wellness.

When working with North Star, the students and I learned how traditional Indigenous teachings of connecting to the land support all other wellness lessons in an ethnically diverse class.

North Star: Connecting to the land helps us maintain good Mental health, while also maintaining Physical, Emotional, and Spiritual health. It reminds us that the Earth is the source of our food and water. From the beginning of the pandemic, taking care of myself has meant smoking my pipe out on the land near the water, walking in my Ancestral territories, and harvesting the medicines I carry. Walking on the land of my Ancestors feels like a constant dialogue or prayer. It helps me to live a good life or, as we say in Anishinaabemowin, Mino Pimatisiwin.

Being outside also supports the health of the students I teach. "The constant interaction with the land, by knowing it with all five senses, guides individuals and provides what is needed to lie in harmony with the environment, with each other, and with oneself. The reciprocal and dialogic relationship with nature provides not only the material needs but also the ethical, moral, and spiritual underpinnings of living a good life" (Radu et al., 2014, p. 93). Our sacred ceremonies are situated outside in nature. Depending on the territory, we build our teaching and initiation lodges from the surrounding environment. I know what these outdoor classrooms do for me and my spirit, so now my lessons take place outside as much as possible. It is our job to support students in their mental health as well as maintain our own. I teach students to embrace nature and the world around them as a dear relative. When we see the land and water in this way, then we will stand up and protect it because it is sacred.

Having a positive relationship with the Earth helps us develop a deep, meaningful relationship with ourselves within the Sacred Hoop. It takes relationships of all kinds to keep our Sacred Hoop in balance. "It is our nature to be whole and to be together. We are born into a circle of family, community, living creatures, and the land" (Wilson, 2015, p. 197). Indigenous Peoples understand that true healing comes from a place of deep knowing and deep listening.

Recently, I have taken classes out to the Bannock Point Petroforms—in my language, Manitou Ahbee. One time, after spending the day sharing the significance of our sacred teaching place, I went home and slept. In a vivid dream, I was told to go and gather Grandparent rocks and take them to the schools I was working in, to share lessons about the teachings and stories of the Anishinaabe people. These lessons, which we conducted outside with Monika's class, allowed experiential and hands-on learning to take place. We told stories using the Grandparent rocks. The students used the rocks to create their own stories. We worked together creatively, building rock formations and sharing stories. This gave us a chance to learn from the land and practise deep listening. The experience was powerful for students and staff alike.

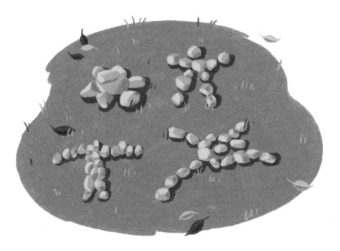

Reflect and Respond
- Walk to a quiet area with your students or family and sit by yourself. Try to quiet your body. Write down all the things you feel—Physical, Emotional, Mental, and Spiritual. What do you see, smell, hear, and touch? What do you feel in your spirit? Take time to connect with everything around you.
- Take a moment to find a place near a body of water. With your students or family, take time to sketch the pond and colour it. Do not rush. Observe and enjoy everything you see, smell, hear, and touch.

- Is there something that you are now aware of that you weren't before? Write about what you are now aware of and now grateful for.
- Take turns to share any awareness or gratitude that you feel, always remembering that each person has the right to pass if they choose not to share in this moment.

Closing Thoughts

In this chapter, we have shared wellness practices we have experienced through our relationships with students, ourselves, each other, and the land. We each shared our perspectives and stories of well-being as teachers. Class wellness practices that have benefited our students have also shaped our understanding of our personal wellness, which is tied to the land we live on. Each strategy we have used, such as Talking Circles, mindfulness, honesty, and connecting to the land, all support us in our wellness journey when working in the classroom. These practices have a ripple effect that benefits the environment in which we work. We have woven wellness into our everyday teaching lives. We hope these practices can be part of your wellness journey.

References and Further Reading

Brown, B. (2017). *Braving the wilderness: The quest for true belonging and the courage to stand alone.* Random House.

Brown, B. (Host). (2021, May 5). Trauma, resilience, and healing with Oprah Winfrey and Dr. Bruce D. Perry [Audio podcast episode]. In *Brené Brown.* https://brenebrown.com/podcast/brene-with-oprah-winfrey-and-dr-bruce-d-perry-on-trauma-resilience-and-healing/

Garcia, S. N. (n.d.). How SEL helps you as a teacher. Retrieved May 1, 2021, from https://www.understood.org/articles/en/how-sel-helps-you-as-a-teacher

Guarding Minds at Work. (2020). *Know the psychosocial factors.* https://www.guardingmindsatwork.ca/about/about-psychosocial-factors

Kabat-Zinn, J. (1990). *Full catastrophe living: Using the wisdom of your body and mind to face stress, pain, and illness.* Bantam Dell.

Katz, J. (2012). *Teaching to diversity: The three-block model of universal design for learning.* Portage & Main Press.

Katz, J., & Lamoureux, K. (2018). *Ensouling our schools: A universally designed framework for mental health, well-being, and reconciliation.* Portage & Main Press.

Linklater, R. (2014). *Decolonizing trauma work: Indigenous stories and strategies.* Fernwood.

McGonigal, K. (2012). *The willpower instinct: How self-control works, why it matters, and what you can do to get more of it.* Penguin Group.

Radu, I., House, L., & Pashagumskum, E. (2014). Land, life, and knowledge in Chisasibi: Intergenerational healing in the bush. *Decolonization: Indigeneity, Education & Society, 3*(3), 86–105.

Wilson, A. (2015). Our coming in stories: Cree identity, body sovereignty and gender self-determination. *Journal of Global Indigeneity, 1*(1), Article 4.

Chapter 11

Thank You for Being a Friend

A Story of Collegial Support

Kelsey McDonald

Kelsey McDonald's career in public education spans 20-plus years as classroom teacher, resource teacher, school counsellor, and principal. Most recently, she was seconded as the Provincial Consultant for Guidance and Counselling with the Inclusion Support Branch of Manitoba's Department of Education. Having professional experiences from a variety of vantage points has provided Kelsey with a unique perspective on our educational systems. Kelsey holds a BEd and a PBDE from the University of Manitoba, where she is currently enrolled in the MEd Counselling Psychology program. She lives in Winnipeg with her husband, Scott, and sons, Owen and Griffin.

Through my 20-plus years in education, there have been many wonderful experiences made better by being surrounded by caring, compassionate, dedicated teachers. There have also been some very lonely, difficult times in my career that were made better by having the support of those same colleagues. This is the story of my journey to self-awareness, self-compassion, self-acceptance, and learning when to accept support.

I was hired for my first teaching job in mid-September. The class had 32 students, many with complex learning needs. Because of the school's at-risk status, rather than hire an educational assistant to support the current classroom teacher, the school division approved the hire of an additional teacher. The class would be split into two, and I would take on 16 students.

In short, I was not prepared with the skills this job required. From the very first day, I was completely overwhelmed by the challenges in the class. It quickly became clear that, if I was going to survive the year, I was going to need some help. Despite my attempts to feign competence, it was also clear to my principal that I needed help. And thank goodness, because she sent help. Sherry, the school counsellor, was engaged to be my mentor.

Sherry showed up for me and my students. She spent time in my classroom nearly every day. She took me under her wing and taught me the things I didn't learn at university. Her approach was gentle, patient, and compassionate. She helped me to understand that it was okay if we didn't get through all the lessons I had planned for the day. She modelled calm. She allowed me to step out of the room for a minute (or 10) to collect myself when needed. She spent that whole year showing me how to be the teacher that these children needed me to be.

Paying It Forward

Sherry inspired me so much that, during my third year as a teacher, I returned to university to begin earning the credentials to become a school counsellor. I finished my counselling courses while I was on maternity leave (such a bad idea!). After one more year in the classroom, I accepted a transfer to another school to begin my first job as a school counsellor.

Of course, school counsellors provide direct service to students, but a big part of that role is also supporting the staff. Sherry supported my students by supporting me to develop my capacity as a teacher. Thanks to Sherry's mentorship, I had the opportunity to emulate her approach with teachers while I was a school counsellor.

Employees feel that organizations care when they support growth and development, skill acquisition, and career development. This can directly improve employee well-being. It has been shown to increase goal commitment, organizational commitment, and job satisfaction (Guarding Minds at Work, 2020). This was my experience, and it took me down a similar path of mentorship. When I met Claire, she was a first-year teacher who had been assigned an especially challenging group of students. This class of children had tested their previous teacher, who was a skilled and seasoned veteran. I knew that I needed to start building a relationship with Claire right away. She was going to need a lot of support to meet the needs of her students in the year to come.

Claire and I met in August, discussed the needs of the class, and came up with a preliminary plan to use while we each got to know her students. Claire, naturally, wanted some time and space to get acquainted with her class and establish routines on her own. For now, she wanted my role to be with the individual students who were identified as needing additional support. I let her know that I would remain available for whole-class support, and we planned a time in mid-September to touch base about how things were going.

Unfortunately, Claire didn't even get through her first day of teaching without incident. Children who were experiencing emotional and behavioural difficulties demonstrated their distress daily. Those students who witnessed their classmates' difficulties were equally as distressed. Recess often ended in the office. The parent phone calls, emails, and meetings never ended.

Claire and I met often to debrief incidents, revise plans, and strategize about how to get parental support. But she wasn't yet comfortable inviting me to join her in the classroom. I could see Claire's confidence was being depleted. That old saying, "It takes one to know one," came to mind often. The parallels to my first year were uncanny. Claire was giving everything she had, yet still felt like it wasn't enough. I wanted to be worthy of her trust. I knew, from experience, how important it was to have a colleague with whom you could be completely open in meeting the kinds of challenges Claire faced.

So I shared my first-year story and all its shame-filled moments. I told Claire how I raised my voice at my students because of my frustration, and the guilt that followed. I told her about the crying jags in the staff washroom at recess and the terrible, overwhelming sense of failure that permeated my days. Then I shared with Claire how it came to be that Sherry had arrived in my classroom, and how having that support had helped me through the year. That simple act of sharing my story was enough for Claire to accept my invitation for support.

 As an Indigenous person, when I am working with new counsellors or social workers or training staff on how to work with Indigenous Peoples, I tell them to make a connection and build a relationship with people. You need to share some of your story, your struggles, your life. People will respect you more.

> Do not think you have to approach this work in a way that is overly professional, remaining unattached, clinical, and cold. When you share your pain, the people you are trying to build a relationship with, or help, will feel that this comes from your heart and will be more able to be trusting and open to you and willing to share what is going on in their life.—*Elder Kipling*

As fall became winter, I spent much of my days physically present in the classroom. I was supporting the students who were identified as needing additional support or working behind the scenes to access other resources for Claire's class. We brought in specialists to consult and support whole-class programming. We made referrals to clinical services for individual students and their families and created individualized education plans where appropriate. We obtained emergency funding to have a full-time educational assistant in the classroom. As winter wore on, things were slowly improving in the classroom, but Claire was visibly languishing. She stopped coming to the staff room to socialize at lunch. She looked tired, was suffering from regular headaches, and had started to miss work on occasion. My concern for Claire had increased.

After an especially difficult parent meeting, which lasted until after 6 pm, Claire confided in me that she wasn't sleeping. She couldn't stop worrying about her students and her perceived shortcomings as a teacher. I asked Claire if she was aware of the professional counselling help available to teachers through our employee assistance plan benefits. She concluded that it might be time to widen her circle of support.

By the time spring had sprung, Claire was seeing her counsellor regularly. Together they were working on the skills of "leaving work at work" and adding joy back to her days. At the same time, Claire was beginning to see the impact that her efforts were having on her students. She came back to the staff room at lunch. There she made social connections with other staff members who helped her to find humour in some of the situations that transpired within a day.

As the year wound down, Claire knew that she had done the best she could to support her students and was able to recognize the ways she had helped them grow. Most importantly, she was proud of the teacher she was becoming and was looking toward the next school year with optimism. I'm happy to share that Claire now works in a role where she provides mentorship and support to other teachers, paying it forward within our profession.

Taking on the Principalship

Years later, I transitioned into a principalship. Most of the feedback I got about my choice to take on the role of principal, from colleagues and others, was that I was likely biting off more than I could chew by taking on so much responsibility. You see, at the time, my sons were five and nine. They attended different schools and before-and-after programs at different daycares. In addition, my husband, Scott, is a shift worker. Like so many things in this life, it is only through lived experience that one truly appreciates the impact such a variable makes. In short, shift work complicates family life. It needed to be a factor in my decision to work in a role that increased my commitments beyond the school day.

Despite the doubt others expressed, I believed in myself and knew I could make it work. We were also fortunate to have three sets of grandparents who were able to step in and help when there were conflicts with evening activities. So I left school every day with a bag of unfinished work and put on my mom hat. After dinner was prepared, lunches were packed, activities attended, and kids were asleep, out came the bag o' work.

I felt accomplished, and I was proud that I was filling both roles successfully. It was challenging and exhilarating. It was also exhausting. For a few years, I was fuelled by adrenalin and the satisfaction that came from leading a team of dedicated professionals who were committed to their students and their own continuous professional growth. I also had a group of "princi-pals" to lament with on a Friday night here and there, and that relief was enough to keep me going.

Until it wasn't. One particularly difficult school year had me wondering how sustainable it was to continue in the principalship. That year we had a student who was in crisis, and that one individual's actions had far-reaching impacts on the well-being of the students and staff alike. For an extended period that year, for reasons I won't get into, I spent a vast amount of the school day providing one-on-one support to this student.

As a result, I was often working into the wee hours to stay on top of my responsibilities. After the rollercoaster of my workday, I was tired but wired. I wasn't sleeping well, and I couldn't stop worrying about the situation. My worries about the impact of this student's behaviour on the other children and my staff monopolized my thoughts. I was stuck in the unfortunate position of knowing both that I was doing everything within my control and that it was insufficient. Once again, I found myself feeling like I was failing professionally.

 Falling back into old habits and not being mindful of our own stress and wellness is always a concern. We must have people in place who can support us, even when we are thinking things are going well. As an Indigenous person, I use my belief in daily prayer, reflection, time on the land, and working with spiritual things to relax my mind, spirit, body, and emotions. At the same time, I always make sure I have a support person to connect with.—*Elder Kipling*

On top of that, it was getting increasingly difficult to keep my mom guilt in check. I was getting home later and later into the evening and was often the last parent to arrive for daycare pickup. When I got home, I was cranky and preoccupied. My laptop was my constant companion during the boys' evening activities. My white-knuckle motto, "just get through to July," was of absolutely no comfort in February.

When summer finally did arrive, I was completely drained. I spent the first two weeks of vacation taking respite on the beach, more or less comatose and very grateful to have a summer family of lake friends whose generosity allowed my kids to be oblivious to my stupor. After I had come down, I spent the rest of July cherishing the relaxed pace of lake life. It was the balm I needed to show up smiling at school in August.

The following year continued to be challenging. Scott had recently been promoted, and his father was having serious health issues. Between his increased responsibilities at work and supporting his parents, he was less available at home. At the same time, the other two sets of grandparents had both moved away from our city. Our village for raising our kids was becoming incredibly small, and I found it increasingly difficult to do a good job both at work and at home. The concept of work-life balance was laughable. Scott and I were both just getting by. We knew we couldn't sustain this pace.

For the first time, I began to vocalize to someone other than Scott that I was feeling the need for a change. Simply put, I was spreading myself too thin. Something had to give. One night, I sat down with "my person," Genevieve, and let it all out. Genevieve also happened to be one of my teachers so she had an intimate understanding of the situation at school. During that conversation, she asked me a question that helped me to shift my perspective: "So, why won't you let the staff help you, you fool? You help them all the time! They can see that you're run off your feet, and they want to be there for you. Let them."

Up to that point, I had been declining offers for help because I felt it wasn't fair to burden my team with my responsibilities. I had signed up to sit in the big chair, not anyone else. But Genevieve's words helped me to begin thinking differently about things. She helped me to realize that my teachers were offering me the gift of their support. They offered not only because they cared for me as an individual, but also because that's what collaborative teams do—they help one another.

And that is how I learned to have the self-awareness and self-compassion to say "Yes, that would be lovely, thank you" when someone offered to help me. I accepted offers to cover the office for a few minutes so I could visit in the staffroom at recess. I accepted an offer to read the riot act to our misbehaving bus riders when I got intercepted by an anxious parent on my way outside.

On one occasion, a teacher who had been working in her classroom long after dismissal noticed that I was still in the office. She stopped by to shoo me out the door because she knew one of my boys had a school concert that evening. Then she noticed the young pumpkin who was my charge; it was after 5 pm and no one had yet arrived to take this student home. A caregiver was on the way to the school to get the child, but my route home was heavy with traffic at this time of day. I would be lucky to get to the concert on time to see my boy on stage. Knowing this, the teacher put down her bags. She took the book I had been reading to the student. In her no-nonsense teacher voice, she told (not asked) me to get going. I welled up with gratitude and ran out the door, making the concert with only moments to spare, in time to see my little guy beaming at me from the stage.

In particular, it was the school counsellor, Kim, who got me through that year. What felt like every evening, once Kim and I both had our kids snuggled in their beds, the two of us spent time on the phone debriefing the day and strategizing for the next. Without that one person with whom I could commiserate, I'm not sure I would have been able to muster the energy to walk into the building each morning and be the leader my team needed me to be.

I could offer more examples of ways that my staff helped me, but I've made my point. There are times when each of us needs help, and acts of kindness and generosity can make a huge impact on the person in need.

I can see in retrospect that when I accepted help from others, I modelled the importance of accepting help. When we model this for others, we give them permission to do the same.

Accepting help is its own kind of strength.
—*Kiera Cass*

Now I work in a role where I spend my days supporting inclusive practices across our province. My job allows me to contribute to the field I love, in ways that feel right to me, both personally and professionally. That right fit in my professional life is one of the cornerstones of my wellness. I could not have arrived at this place without the support of all the colleagues who have been a friend to me over the years. Some have been named in this story, but there are so many more. You know who you are. Thank you, each of you, for being a friend.

Many people will walk in and out of your life,
but only true friends will leave footprints in your heart.
—*Eleanor Roosevelt*

Mental Health Awareness

During the COVID-19 pandemic, there appears to have been a shift in the way society looks at mental health issues. Television commercials promote strategies for wellness, the rich and famous share their struggles, and employers look for ways to support positive mental health in the workplace. There has been a widespread acknowledgement that we need to do a better job of recognizing the interconnectedness of mental and physical health. COVID-19 has highlighted the need for acceptance of this in our society. What seems a reasonable next step is for all Canadians to have a basic level of mental health literacy so that we share a common understanding of what we mean when we speak about mental health.

The Canadian Mental Health Association states that "mental health is not only the avoidance of serious mental illness. Your mental health is affected by numerous factors from your daily life, including the stress of balancing work with your health and relationships" (Canadian Mental Health Association, n.d.). While stress is a normal part of the human experience, each of us will respond in our unique ways. The Mental Health Commission of Canada (MHCC) has created a model that shows how all human beings experience mental health on a continuum, from healthy to ill. (Search for this continuum at <https://www.theworkingmind.ca/>.)

At each stage of our lives, these experiences and circumstances contribute to where we are on the continuum. Some are described as "risk factors" and others are "protective factors" (Kousoulis, 2019, pp. 12–13). The following two graphics show examples of these factors:

Reflect and Respond
- Think about some of the risk factors that you have experienced. How have they affected your mental health?
- Identify some of the protective factors that you experience. How have these helped you build resilience?

Of course, because of our personal experiences and life stories, each of us can relate in some way to these risk factors and protective factors, teachers included. Yet many of our teaching colleagues have suffered in silence. In some sense, there seems to be an unspoken subtext in our profession that, because our roles are to support others, we should not need help ourselves. We have an opportunity to leave this mindset where it belongs, in the past.

What Can You Do to Help Your Fellow Teachers?

"In the context of exposure to significant adversity, resilience is … the capacity of individuals to navigate their way to the psychological, social, cultural, and physical resources that sustain their well-being" (Ungar, 2008). We need to consider the ways that we can build resilience while supporting ourselves, our individual colleagues, and the collective of our colleagues. Even while acknowledging our struggles, we can share our resilience with others.

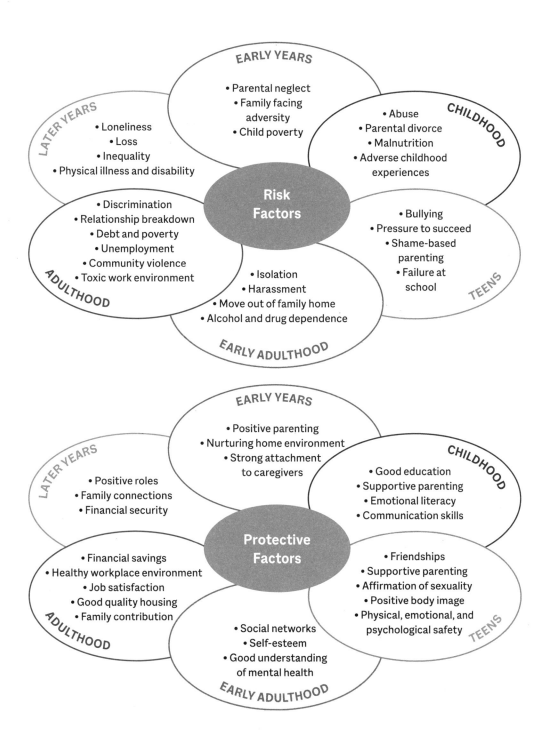

Risk Factors

LATER YEARS
- Loneliness
- Loss
- Inequality
- Physical illness and disability

EARLY YEARS
- Parental neglect
- Family facing adversity
- Child poverty

CHILDHOOD
- Abuse
- Parental divorce
- Malnutrition
- Adverse childhood experiences

ADULTHOOD
- Discrimination
- Relationship breakdown
- Debt and poverty
- Unemployment
- Community violence
- Toxic work environment

TEENS
- Bullying
- Pressure to succeed
- Shame-based parenting
- Failure at school

EARLY ADULTHOOD
- Isolation
- Harassment
- Move out of family home
- Alcohol and drug dependence

Protective Factors

LATER YEARS
- Positive roles
- Family connections
- Financial security

EARLY YEARS
- Positive parenting
- Nurturing home environment
- Strong attachment to caregivers

CHILDHOOD
- Good education
- Supportive parenting
- Emotional literacy
- Communication skills

ADULTHOOD
- Financial savings
- Healthy workplace environment
- Job satisfaction
- Good quality housing
- Family contribution

TEENS
- Friendships
- Supportive parenting
- Affirmation of sexuality
- Positive body image
- Physical, emotional, and psychological safety

EARLY ADULTHOOD
- Social networks
- Self-esteem
- Good understanding of mental health

There is no doubt that school staff need to feel support, not only professionally, but also personally. This means creating a work environment where coworkers and supervisors understand the significance of colleagues' well-being and support them appropriately during times of success and challenge. In chapter 13, there is a review of 13 psychosocial factors that protect employee mental health, as identified in the National Standard of Canada for Psychological Health and Safety in the Workplace. There is much that we can learn from paying attention to these factors, both as leaders and as colleagues. This is echoed by the EdCan Network, which created Well at Work to support education leaders to develop and implement system-wide strategies to improve K to 12 workplace well-being for the long term. The research is clear that when we invest in teacher well-being, we are investing in a healthy school community (EdCan Network, 2022).

Self-Care: The Importance of Healthy Individuals

Early in my first principalship, a small team of staff from our school had the opportunity to participate as observers in a residency with educational leader Regie Routman. I had read a number of her books ahead of time, but the experience of observing her teach students in a room full of educators was what helped me to understand her messages. One such teaching is Routman's emphatic belief that if we are to be truly excellent inside the classroom, we need to lead full, meaningful lives outside of the classroom (Routman, as cited in Ferlazzo, 2018). My unexpected takeaway from this professional development opportunity was a deeper appreciation of the ways we shortchange everyone when we run ourselves into the ground in the name of our work. There tends to be a culture of teacher martyrdom, and this is hurting our profession (Fan, 2021). Our students, our colleagues, and our schools are better for it when we prioritize our well-being.

One emerging idea worthy of considering for your own self-care is an annual mental health checkup:

> Once a year, you visit your medical doctor for an annual checkup to check in on your physical health and for the prevention and early detection of disease. However, when it comes to mental health, many of us do not consider seeing a doctor or professional about our mental health unless we felt there was something drastically wrong. This may be part of the problem why so many Canadians are experiencing mental health challenges. They are missing the

opportunity for early intervention. Mental health, like our physical health, can benefit from a proactive mental health checkup to provide information about our status and help us make a plan to influence our actions and change our behaviour. (Howatt, 2019)

The adage "an ounce of prevention" comes to mind here. We are fortunate to work in a field where we have access to mental health professionals, through employee assistance programs or our extended health benefits. What better way to care for ourselves than by having a screening for our mental health each year?

Reflect and Respond
- How would you fare on a mental health checkup today? You might want to complete the MHCC self-check described earlier: <https://theworkingmind.ca/continuum-self-check>.
- In what ways are you demonstrating positive mental health?
- In what ways are you experiencing challenges to your mental health?

School Culture: We Each Play a Role

School culture is an interesting concept to capture; it is ubiquitous and intangible. School culture can be defined as "the guiding beliefs and values evident in the way a school operates" (Fullan, 2007). The term can be used to encompass all the attitudes, expected behaviours, and values that have an impact on how the school functions. Here we'll focus on the ways teachers interact with one another and contribute to or detract from a healthy school culture. Every day, we each arrive at work with an opportunity to make the day a little better for our colleagues. Here are a few things each of us can try to do to promote workplace wellness in our school communities:

Normalize "Not Okay" Days: The Canadian Mental Health Association (CMHA) has launched Not Myself Today, a support for employers to help transform mental health at work. According to the CHMA (2019), 95 percent of employees use another reason when they take time away from work for mental health. This initiative provides help by providing all employees with tools to contribute to a more healthful workplace culture. Consider sharing the CMHA four-minute video "Not Myself Today" with your principal and begin the "It's okay to not be okay" conversation (<https://www.notmyselftoday.ca>).

Often, when we are not at our best, putting on a brave face is the hardest part of coming to school. Let's work together to change the culture in schools of having to be "okay" all the time. The next time you are having a down day and a colleague asks, "How are you?" consider an honest reply by taking the courageous step of saying, "I'm not myself today." Our choices and actions as individuals have a great impact on the culture in our schools; you can help normalize "not okay" days.

Choose Your Words Carefully: To help break down mental health stigma, we need to be aware of the language we use. In education, we've learned how to support inclusion by using respectful language to discuss a wide array of diversity: religious, cultural, ability, socioeconomic, gender, and more. Let's work together to expand that respect to the language we use to talk about mental health. When we casually toss about words like "crazy" or "nuts" to describe ourselves or others, we are perpetuating the stereotypes that cause some teachers who struggle to do so silently. Using respectful language is a step toward a more inclusive world. The MHCC has developed a resource to help our understanding of how language matters. The Language Matters "cheat sheet" was created to help us choose respectful and empowering language (MHCC, 2022).

Learn Together: A wide variety of professional development opportunities can support your school staff to enhance mental health literacy. Advocate for this to improve the culture of your workplace. It will benefit both staff and students. Below are some of the national organizations that support these efforts. Explore the supports that are available in your community.

- Canadian Mental Health Association has a variety of programs to support workplace mental health: <https://cmha.ca/programs-services/workplace-mental-health>.
- Canadian Red Cross: <https://www.redcross.ca/training-and-certification/course-descriptions/psychological-first-aid-courses/psychological-first-aid>.
- Mental Health Commission of Canada: <https://www.mentalhealthcommission.ca/English>.

Walk the Walk: We spend a lot of school time teaching our students about kindness, diversity, and inclusion. Those are the cornerstones of a safe and caring learning environment for all. We also need to ensure that inclusion is intentionally visible when we walk into the staff room. We must create a community in our staff room, hallways, workshops, and staff meetings. Teaching can be isolating work. We are alone with our students most of the day, so collegiality is paramount to our individual and collective well-being. So, what to do? Try sitting with someone new at lunch; pop into a colleague's classroom, someone you haven't yet gotten to know; be generous with compliments. You'll feel good about being inclusive and doing your part to support a healthy school culture. We talk the talk to our students. We need to walk the walk and model this for our students by treating all our colleagues with kindness, dignity, and respect.

Closing Thoughts

Regardless of the culture of your school or the measures put in place to enhance workplace wellness, there will be times when you notice that an individual colleague needs more support. Examples of ways that we can help our colleagues have been sprinkled throughout this chapter. But what can you do when those things aren't enough? "Our relationships [at work] are intimate whether we want it that way or not, so when a colleague is suffering in some way, … it must be recognized. The best way to do that will depend on your relationship with the coworker" (Lucy Bichsel, as cited in Luckwaldt, 2019).

If the colleague is also a friend, you can initiate a conversation gently and compassionately to guide that colleague to access resources or professional help. If the relationship is strictly collegial, this can be a difficult decision. Your actions will depend on the context and severity of the situation. If you have significant concerns, you may wish to confidentially share them with your principal, who can help connect the individual with support. Or you may choose to have a confidential consultation with your local teachers' association representative or someone in human resources (both while keeping your colleague anonymous) about appropriate ways to offer your support. To be clear, this is not about "telling on a teacher." This is about wanting our colleagues—and ourselves—to have the support we all need to be well both in and out of our work. Chapter 12, "The Principal's Principles," explores this topic in more detail by outlining a process to follow when colleagues are struggling.

In the end, we must all recognize that we have a responsibility to ourselves and our colleagues. We must take care of ourselves and each other. Self-care is work and it requires intentional effort. How do we, as teachers, support one another to prioritize self-care and improve the cultures in our workplaces?

We don't control the pressures of the systems in which we work. But we can do the things that are within our power, to care for ourselves and to contribute to creating a school culture that promotes positive mental health. And that means understanding the issues, acting, and being a friend.

Reflect and Respond

Schools with healthy cultures are a pleasure to work in. If your workplace is less so, you may feel like there is not much one individual can do to make a change. Look for others who will be your allies in the goal of making your school a more inclusive, healthy workplace, and live your ethics together.

- To learn more about ending discrimination related to mental health, see the Bring Change to Mind website: <https://bringchange2mind.org>.
- What actions can you take, today? Is there another colleague to whom you could be more of a friend?
- To learn more about promoting pro-social behaviour among adults, review the resources on the CASEL: Guide to Schoolwide SEL website: <https://schoolguide.casel.org/focus-area-2/overview/>.
- How can you advocate for intentional change, to help your school team consciously improve their interactions with one another? What can you ask of your principal?
- What action will you take as an individual to "be the change" after reading this chapter?

References and Further Reading

Bring Change to Mind. (n.d.). *Choose your words*. Retrieved March 2021, from https://bringchange2mind.org/talk/choose-your-words/

Canadian Mental Health Association (CMHA). (n.d.). *Mental health* [Brochure]. Retrieved May 17, 2021, from https://cmha.ca/document-category/mental-health

Canadian Mental Health Association National. (2019, April 23). *Not myself today* [Video, 2:25]. YouTube. https://www.youtube.com/watch?v=qaCpukxBM-0

Collaborative for Academic, Social, and Emotional Learning. (n.d.). *The CASEL guide to schoolwide SEL*. Retrieved April 2021, from https://schoolguide.casel.org/

EdCan Network. (2022). *What is "Well at Work"?* Well at work. https://k12wellatwork.ca/

Fan, R. (2021, April 30). Teaching is not martyrdom. *Psychology Today*. https://www.psychologytoday.com/ca/blog/social-emotional-learning-teachers/202104/teaching-is-not-martyrdom

Ferlazzo, L. (2018, June 14). Author interview with Regie Routman: "Literacy Essentials." *EducationWeek*. https://www.edweek.org/teaching-learning/opinion-author-interview-with-regie-routman-literacy-essentials/2018/06

Fullan, M. (2007). *The new meaning of educational change* (4th ed.). Teachers College Press. https://michaelfullan.ca/books/new-meaning-educational-change/

Guarding Minds at Work. (2020). *Know the psychosocial factors*. https://www.guardingmindsatwork.ca/about/about-psychosocial-factors.

———. (2022). *Workplace strategies for mental health*. https://www.workplacestrategiesformentalhealth.com/resources/guarding-minds-at-work-survey-statements.

Howatt, B. (2019, January 30). Why you need to do an annual mental health check up. *The Globe and Mail*. https://www.theglobeandmail.com/business/careers/workplace-award/article-why-you-need-to-do-an-annual-mental-health-check-up/

Kolappa, K., Henderson, D. C., & Kishore, S. P. (2013, January 1). No physical health without mental health: Lessons unlearned? *Bulletin of the World Health Organization*, *91*(1), 3–3A. doi:10.2471/BLT.12.115063

Kousoulis, D. (2019). *Prevention and mental health: Understanding the evidence so that we can address the greatest health challenge of our times*. Mental Health Foundation. https://www.mentalhealth.org.uk/sites/default/files/2022-06/MHF-Prevention-report-2019.pdf

Luckwaldt, J. H. (2019, May 10). *How to support your coworker who's dealing with mental health issues*. Payscale. https://www.payscale.com/career-news/2019/05/how-to-support-your-coworker-whos-dealing-with-mental-health-issues

Mental Health Commission of Canada (MHCC). (2021). *Continuum self check.* https://theworkingmind.ca/continuum-self-check

———. (2022). *Language matters.* https://www.mentalhealthcommission.ca/wp-content/uploads/drupal/2020-08/language_matters_cheat_sheet_eng.pdf

Ungar, M. (2008). Resilience across cultures [Research note]. *British Journal of Social Work, 38*(2), 218–35. https://doi.org/10.1093/bjsw/bcl343

Chapter 12

The Principal's Principles
School Leadership for Staff Wellness

Sandra Pacheco Melo

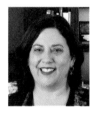

Sandra Pacheco Melo, PBDE, MEd, has been an educator for more than 28 years in the public school system in Manitoba. She is currently principal at a French immersion early years school. Sandra speaks Portuguese, English, and French. She is a former classroom, resource, and divisional support teacher in K to 12. Sandra lives with her husband, John, and daughters Mattias and Allysia.

Imagine coming into work after not sleeping all night because you were unable to shut off the brain that insisted that sleep was your enemy. The brain that could not shut off because it played and replayed conversations that happened at school.

> "Sandra, I'm falling apart. My child is suffering from extreme anxiety; I am struggling to get through a lesson with my students because I stayed up with him last night. Can I take a sick day tomorrow to get some rest?"
>
> "Should we send Braxton home? He is sick but I know his parents can't miss any more work to get him from school. They could lose their jobs. But what if it's contagious?"
>
> "Sandra, the first stall in the bathroom is locked and it's a mess. Who is going to clean it? The custodian is gone for the day and the nighttime cleaner does not start until 4 pm."

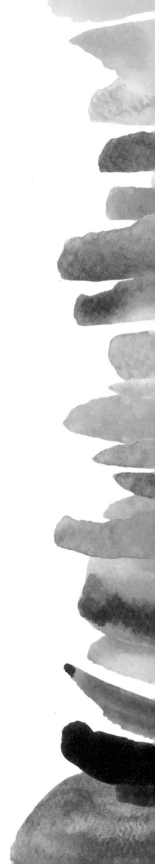

Let's excavate the routine life of a school leader in our current scenario, as educators during a pandemic. While this book is not about supporting mental wellness during a worldwide health crisis, it is no secret that we have lived through the most challenging school years in recent history. For many teachers and school leaders, the challenges of keeping themselves physically and mentally healthy were greater than the trials of instructing the students.

These challenges increased exponentially for school leaders, especially as attendance waned. As a principal of an elementary school, I found that, at times, they seemed to outweigh the joy that I once found in coming to work. That feeling of knowing that nothing was getting better, and we had months ahead of more of the same, made leading in this otherwise vibrant community tough! It was more than the pandemic stressors. It was the daily lives, exhaustion, and demands of the educators that had me, as a leader, concerned about staff well-being.

I thought back to some of my mentors and imagined what they would say at a time like this. I had to make the conscious decision to lace up my shoes and lead—lead from the heart and the head. My internal voice said, "Chin up! If you are not the calm in the chaos, then who is?" I concentrated my efforts as a leader on keeping the staff safe, healthy, happy, calm, and focused on joy, gratitude, and strength. I faced many daily stressors in trying to run a school without impeding student learning or negatively affecting the staff's emotional and physical well-being.

Canadian child psychologist Dr Jody Carrington suggests that school leaders need to create a culture "where relationship knows no hierarchy" (2020, p. 149). In other words, as the leader, you need to create an environment in which relationships can flourish between students, families, and staff. Leaders need to promote workplace wellness to stay connected, healthy, and motivated. Moreover, they need to support the mental health of staff as much as that of students, all while keeping themselves healthy too. This is an immense challenge and responsibility. Yet it can be incredibly rewarding and is necessary to clear the way for a thriving school and community.

So how does a principal lead for mental wellness? Once I had decided that my role was to be a strong and solid foundation for my staff, I resolved to lead a well school with a focus on joy, gratitude, mindfulness, and laughter.

 For all the heartbreak we have faced as Indigenous Peoples, we have always maintained one strength: laughter! When working hard, playing, or crying with one another, we like to tease and joke. We have a deep understanding that no matter how tough a situation becomes, we can still find laughter and joy in the chaos. Laughter is healing. As Anishinaabe People, we have seven natural Healing Ways: yelling, crying, shaking, yawning, talking, sweating, and laughing. We often experience all seven Healing Ways at sacred ceremonies in Sweat Lodges. There we purge toxins and let go of things that no longer serve us.—*North Star*

Servant Leadership and Positive Psychology: The Bricks and Mortar of a Mentally Well School

If you have ever experienced your own cycle of burnout, or observed stress, anxiety, and burnout in your staff, you may be wondering about prevention and how to be proactive as a leader in fostering mental well-being in your school community. Research indicates that servant leadership has a positive effect in reducing emotional exhaustion, depersonalization, and burnout for both the leader (and aspiring leaders as well) and their staff (Rivkin et al., 2014).

Principals who model servant leadership can increase others' effectiveness and a desire to build and maintain a healthy school community. This can have a positive impact on their students, colleagues, and parents. A servant-leader's words, actions, and relationships have wide-reaching ramifications and positive outcomes for all involved. Maintaining a well school, therefore, becomes a vital part of the principal's role. As mentioned in chapter 1, "The Evolution of *Teacher, Take Care*," research indicates that there are 10 characteristics that servant-leaders exhibit, and these traits have a direct impact on wellness. These are listening, empathy, healing, awareness, persuasion, conceptualization, foresight, stewardship, commitment to growth, and community building (Spears, 2018). However, if you are already feeling stressed or burned out, adopting all of the characteristics of servant leadership may seem like a lot to take on. We invite you to be curious, to explore some of these ideas, and not feel that you have to take it all on your shoulders at once.

Some of these characteristics may take priority at different times. In my experience, the characteristics directly connected to the five building blocks of the PERMAH theory of well-being (as discussed in chapters 2 and 8) are integral to the maintenance of a well school. This model is grounded in the field of positive psychology, which is the scientific study of the factors that enable individuals and communities to flourish. The school community includes all types of individuals—students, staff, and families—in the broadest sense of the term. It is a microcosm of the larger community, which includes the school district and the province, or the macrocosm. According to positive psychology, the microcosm, in this case the school, needs to be well and flourish in relation to all five of the building blocks of the PERMAH model. The H, the building block of health, focuses on the significant role that physical health plays in overall well-being. As identified and described in chapter 2, "Permission to Be Well," the building blocks are:

- Positive Emotion
- Engagement
- Relationships
- Meaning
- Accomplishment
- Health

In chapter 2, the focus of PERMAH is on individual wellness. However, these components can also be used to help to frame how a well school community functions. Specifically, these elements help to sustain wellness during critical times, such as during a pandemic.

Servant leadership and positive psychology are the bricks and mortar of leading a well school and can be a foundation for workplace wellness. By demonstrating the characteristics of servant leadership and combining them with a focus on the building blocks of PERMAH, the leader has a framework that can withstand the challenges that arise in the school community. Within this framework, and with intentional attention to the overall well-being of personnel, we can create safe and healthy spaces for staff. School can be a workplace where psychological health and safety are fostered, where staff can be vulnerable, grow, and sustain wellness in difficult situations.

 Leading a well school is similar to sustaining a healthy community. Our animal teacher is the Wolf who, through their leadership of the pack, shows us how to lead. Our leaders have to be selfless in their immense undertaking. In sustaining a healthy community, the leaders of the pack lead by feeding the pack before they feed themselves. The Elders and babies eat first. Ultimately, in taking care of the community, the leaders are ensuring their own survival as well as the future survival of the pack.—*North Star*

Reflect and Respond

Whether you are a formal or informal leader in your school, think about the individual building blocks of PERMAH.

- How do you foster each of these in your school community? Record specific examples of how you have practised PERMAH in your school.

Here are some examples:

- *Positive Emotion:* Gratitude, forgiveness, savouring, mindfulness, hope, optimism
- *Engagement:* Being challenged and rewarded by your work and goals
- *Relationships:* Connecting, cultivating positive relationships, trusting, being authentic
- *Meaning:* Connecting to something larger than ourselves, sense of purpose, making meaning
- *Accomplishment:* Believing in ourselves, pursuing goals, reaching for our personal best
- *Health:* Taking care of our bodies and minds, physical well-being

Characteristics of a Servant-Leader

Practising the traits of servant leadership enables principals to support others, and themselves, so that they can flourish intellectually and emotionally. In this way, servant leadership sets the groundwork for wellness, from the individual to the school, to the larger educational system. Here's a review of these traits, as introduced in chapter 1, "The Evolution of *Teacher, Take Care*":

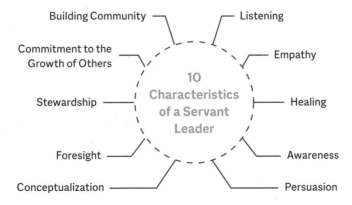

The chart below presents these 10 characteristics of servant-leaders, along with examples of their impact on educator wellness.

Servant Leadership in Action		
Trait	What does it look like in action?	How does it support wellness in others?
Listening	Servant-leaders demonstrate effective communication skills by listening attentively to others.	Being listened to is empowering and encourages us to share our feelings. This, in turn, validates the importance of our wellness.
Empathy	A good servant-leader strives to understand, support, and empathize with others.	Empathy helps to develop positive relationships, which are critical to personal and organizational wellness.
Healing	Servant-leaders have the ability to heal themselves and others, which enables people and systems to overcome problems and challenges.	A positive environment, where individuals are encouraged to heal and flourish, creates a sense of wellness.
Awareness	Servant-leaders take the time to be introspective about their beliefs and actions.	Self-awareness is closely tied to mindfulness, which is a central foundation of well-being and well-becoming.
Persuasion	A servant-leader will effectively persuade others, not by attempting to coerce them, but instead by building consensus.	When individuals believe that their voice matters, they feel empowered, which leads to a sense of agency and self-confidence, both of which are critical components of wellness.
Conceptualization	Servant-leaders who conceptualize have a big-picture perspective and vision for future goals.	Having the ability to dream, hope, and set goals for the future is a component of self-awareness and positive mental health.

Servant Leadership in Action		
Foresight	Servant-leaders with foresight have thought through the possible outcomes of a scenario and consider current realities as well as potential consequences in order to make the best decisions possible.	Foresight allows us to explore decisions and actions to better envision consequences. This offers us self-efficacy, in that we believe that we can influence the conditions that affect our lives, including personal wellness.
Stewardship	Servant-leaders are stewards; their goals and actions are not self-serving, but for the greater good of an organization and society as whole.	A workplace steward fosters a sense of belonging and acknowledgement by ensuring that the needs of others are met, including social-emotional needs.
Commitment to the growth of others	Servant-leaders are committed to the individual growth of human beings and will do everything they can to nurture others.	Being supported and nurtured in personal and professional growth is key to everyone's well-being.
Building community	A servant-leader seeks ways to build community.	Building community fosters a sense of belonging that has a positive effect on individuals' mental health. People thrive in environments where they engage with one another, where everyone feels wanted and is treated as a valuable, capable, and responsible member of the community.

Sources: Crippen, 2005; Crippen, 2010; Hu et al., 2020; Rivkin et al., 2014

Reflect and Respond
- Who, in your life, is a servant-leader?
- How does this person foster wellness in others?

Practical Strategies for Maintaining Wellness

In my experience, explicit and intentional attention to the well-being of the professional school community is one way that leaders can support staff and promote workplace wellness in a proactive manner. I integrate the following activities into staff meetings and professional development days to promote wellness and reflection throughout the school year. (To support a feeling of safety, provide choice. Let staff know that anyone can pass on an activity if they prefer not to participate.)

Picture Your Wellness: This activity is good for connecting to emotions. Randomly choose various pictures to provoke emotions and scatter them all over tables. Ask staff to pick a picture that resonated for them at the time. When someone tells how a picture relates to their mental wellness, they are expressing themselves, making verbal connections to emotions, and connecting to others as they express emotions. As Dr Dan Siegel (n.d.) says, "You gotta name it to tame it."

Our Lives in Photos—Celebrating Joy: Ahead of time, invite staff to send photos to you of joyful times in their lives. The photos are put into a PowerPoint and shared as people are coming into the meeting. This activity encourages you to focus on positives as you are about to enter a difficult meeting or session. Allow staff time to talk to one another about the photos and share with colleagues what brings joy to them. (Source: Sandra Pacheco Melo, Yvonne Perry)

Spirit Buddies Check-in: Provide intentional questions for a well-being check as you enter your monthly staff meetings. For example, provide staff with the question "How was your last week—and if you could make it better, how would you do that?" Staff share their responses in pairs. Personal check-ins with a colleague could allow someone in need to express what is going on. Focus on the second part of the question, which revolves around the positivity and "making things better" aspect. (Source: Katz, 2012)

Sending a Positive Message: Provide each staff member with an index card. They select one other staff member's name from a bag. On the index card, the person writes something positive or gives thanks to the person whose name they drew. They have the option of signing the card or not. They write the name of the person who is receiving the card on the back. Everyone returns the cards to a table, face down. Staff read the messages in private whenever they want or need something positive. In this activity, you intentionally put others first. Thinking of others and reaching out is part of creating a healthy workplace. Focus on positivity, strengths, and gratitude. (Source: Sandra Pacheco Melo, Yvonne Perry)

Gratitude Jar: Make up small mason jars of chocolates for each staff member. Give staff the jar, along with two or three small pieces of paper to write on. Ask staff to write something they are grateful for on the paper. Only when they have given gratitude for something and written it down can they take a treat in exchange from the jar. Each time they add a note, they may take a treat. Focus on gratitude more than once. It takes several intentional moments to have a mindset that focuses on gratitude. Purposefully self-reflecting on what is working or going well in our lives contributes to our wellness. (Source: Sandra Pacheco Melo, Yvonne Perry)

Sensory Mindful Moments: Provide staff with a treat such as a candy cane or cinnamon heart to hold in their mouths for a minute. While they are enjoying the treat, help them be present in the moment by calling attention to the taste, calmness, and quiet. This activity can also be done with a feather to focus on the sense of touch. Or consider providing staff with an opportunity to experience the five senses by naming things that they can see, hear, touch, smell, and taste. Focusing on the senses provides a mindful way to reflect on the moment and be present. It also allows staff to move from stress to calm in an intentional manner. (Source: Keith Macpherson)

Music and Lights: Reduce or dim lighting and play calming instrumental music as staff enter into meetings. Make a deliberate transition to a calming space after a long day. This allows staff to reduce anxiety, sit quietly, chat, and relax, much as we do for our students. (Source: Sandra Pacheco Melo, Yvonne Perry)

A Quiet Reset and Recognition: When gathering for a meeting, take the first full minute for staff to sit quietly, without interruption or anyone asking anything of them. Offer this as a pause to catch their breath and be mindful. As a leader, allow yourself this moment to do the same. At the end of the minute, you might share appreciation for all that staff have given of themselves to get to this point in the day and remind them to take care of themselves for the rest of the day and into the evening or weekend. As part of modelling permission for self-care, let them know that you will try to do the same. (Source: Shannon Gander)

Colouring: Provide staff with pages from adult colouring books to colour during the meeting. In this way, you begin with a calming intention and reduce stress. This allows staff to reduce anxiety, sit quietly, chat, and relax much like what we do for our students. (Source: Monday Mandala <https://mondaymandala.com>)

Wellness Quickwrite: Provide staff with opportunities to reflect on their wellness. This strategy encourages freestyle writing without the stress of expectations for lengthy text. Simply pose a few questions to staff and give them five minutes to write freely. Some sample questions include the following: What are you currently doing for self-care? How would you describe your current sense of well-being? What more might you do for yourself? (Source: Jennifer E. Lawson)

Star Breathing: Have staff draw a star with five points, or provide a pre-drawn star. Teach staff to breathe in slowly for three seconds while tracing the star with their fingers and breathe out slowly for four seconds while continuously tracing the star. Acknowledge that this may be the first quiet moment in a demanding day. This is helpful for being present and gives staff a strategy to use when their emotions are activated. (Source: Shannon Gander)

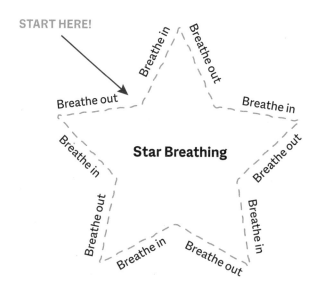

Coupons for Recess Duty: Provide staff with a coupon to use as an exchange for coverage of recess duty. You will cover for them whenever the coupon is asked to be used. Giving staff a break when they decide they need it most can help them to rest, get their bearings, and return to class refreshed. (Source: Sandra Pacheco Melo, Yvonne Perry)

Using activities such as these helps teachers to be mindful of their own wellness and the wellness of those around them. They promote well-being and a culture of taking care, while giving permission to staff to share their successes and challenges with wellness.

Reflect and Respond

Is there an activity or two from the above list that interests you? Write them down for yourself and consider where you might experiment with one of the activities.

Helping Others Who May Be in Crisis

Even though we try to work intentionally and explicitly to keep staff well, a crisis may occur. As educators, we are not all trained in mental health, nor do we have the skills to help someone without external supports. In fact, it is simply not our job to take on the whole issue. Instead, we need to know how to approach a colleague in crisis and begin the process of finding appropriate supports. We need to build our toolkits as leaders to provide support and resources.

One of the most recognized training frameworks in this area is the Mental Health First Aid (MHFA) certification program, researched and developed out of Australia (Kitchener and Jorm, 2002). This program is offered regularly to school staff as well as workers in all other fields. The MHFA program teaches participants how to initially help a person who is facing a mental health challenge or experiencing a mental health crisis. The desired outcome is to increase awareness, increase confidence, and decrease mental health stigma in the workplace and in society.

The MHFA program outlines five basic steps to follow when you believe someone might be unwell and need support. "ALGEE is the framework for having a confident conversation about mental health with family, friends, colleagues, and strangers"

(MHCC, n.d.). The acronym ALGEE spells out the steps to support someone who may be in need.

A	Assess the risk of suicide and/or harm
L	Listen nonjudgmentally
G	Give reassurance
E	Encourage professional support
E	Encourage other supports

These steps are presented only as a precursor to formal training. The MHFA program also explores issues of substance use, depression, anxiety, trauma, and psychotic disorders, as well as crisis interventions for overdose, suicidal behaviour, panic attacks, psychotic episodes, and acute stress reaction.

There are many other approaches and training programs available to individuals, workplaces, and organizations. Another valuable program is the Workplace Mental Health Leadership certificate program (LifeWorks, 2021), which is a leader-focused training opportunity intended to provide mental health professional development for those in supervisory positions who support other employees. The program highlights organizational leadership and emphasizes the importance of demonstrating responsibility and intentional commitment to mentally healthy workplaces. (See the LifeWorks website: <https://lifeworks-learning.com>.) Accessing professional development opportunities like these can help us to grow our own knowledge around mental wellness. It can also provide us with at least a foundation for helping others who may be in crisis. And it helps us to talk more openly about mental health concerns.

 It is imperative that we build a safe, respectful, supportive, and nonjudgmental atmosphere when helping Indigenous families. Many of the mental health issues that arise with parents who live with intergenerational trauma may be present. Crisis training can be very helpful. Calling Child and Family Services should never be the knee-jerk reaction when someone is dealing with anxiety. These traumas are not something that we created. Rather, they were caused by policies created to suppress us as a form of cultural genocide and forced upon us with many catastrophic results.—*North Star*

Look in the Mirror

Being a school leader can be an amazing and rewarding experience. It is also a stressful and complicated job. At times, the duties and responsibilities can be overwhelming.

> Not only are our school principals responsible for maintaining a safe and effective educational atmosphere for students, but they have the added responsibility for developing and coaching a solid team of teachers and administrators and they must be available to parents for any school-related issue that may arise with their student. (Douglas, 2020)

In addition to all of the stressors mentioned above, we must also acknowledge that school leaders may suffer from emotional fatigue, vicarious trauma (empathetically engaging with trauma survivors), post-traumatic stress disorder, interpersonal conflicts, and many other challenges to their own wellness. And this is all while navigating the daily routines of school management, budgets, timetables, difficult student behaviours, and often maintaining the critical role of instructional leader too.

School leaders must be intentional and explicit with their own self-care. They "must not forgo their own wellness in the misguided view that making sacrifices in this regard can possibly result in a healthy workplace or learning environment" (Kowalchuk, 2014).

So what can we do to take care of ourselves? First and foremost, be willing to reach out for our own mental health support just as we would seek medical support for physical ailments.

One valuable resource is the Happiness Lab website (<https://www.happinesslab.fm/>) which includes Psychology of Happiness podcasts by Dr Laurie Santos. In her science-based podcasts she shares insights that can change the way we think about happiness and presents tools we can use to learn to relax and reduce stressors. The Happiness Lab also shares Vex King's "24 Ways to Improve Mental Health" (2018). A few suggestions are asking for help, being outside in nature, making a playlist of feel-good songs, and taking breaks from social media and your phone. These can be incorporated into the life of a school leader, or anyone, for that matter.

Mental wellness relies on the leader seeing the school in its entirety, the macrocosm, the inter-relations—or wahkootowin as my colleague says in chapter 4, "Restoring the Circle." We cannot separate the wellness of our students from the wellness of the teachers, families, and the entire community. It is imperative to remember as leaders that we need to keep relationships at the forefront of every decision we make. As a servant-leader, the relationships you build with others start with the relationship you have with yourself. In essence, you need to care for, listen to, and commit to yourself.

Six Practices to Keep Us Motivated and Well

According to Dr Jody Carrington (2020), there are six go-to practices that we can use to keep us motivated and well. They are not sequential and can be used anytime when we feel drained or overburdened.

- *"Who Matters?"* Ask yourself who, in your world, matters most to you? Who would you want to make proud? Who would you want to impress the most? Dead or alive, who are they? Aim for about five names or so and make a list. Keep this list and think about these people every time you must make a big decision. In big moments, only their opinions matter (p. 178). "The rest don't score."
- *"Choose Joy!"* (p. 179). Joy must be conscious and explicit as well as practised. Joy can be found everywhere if you pay attention to it. Look for it in as many places as possible and, before you know it, you will be finding it everywhere. It takes practice.
- *"Gratitude and Intention"* (p. 181). Try to choose three different things to be grateful for every day. You will notice it will change your breath and relax your body. Intention is a prayer without having to ask anyone for anything. "Setting an intention to focus more on something or someone, to bring awareness to an emotion or a connection with someone or something, will bring that into focus" (p. 183).
- *"Practise the F-Word"* (p. 186). The practice of forgiveness involves offering something positive in return such as empathy, compassion, and understanding toward the person who hurt you. Carrington asserts that true forgiveness is linked to "positive mental health outcomes such as reduced anxiety, a reduction of depression and major psychiatric disorders, fewer physical health symptoms and lower mortality rates" (p. 186).
- *"Collective Effervescence"* (p. 190). Staying connected to your team is of the utmost importance, especially since as educators we are wired to do hard things. In addition, as humans we are "wired for connection," so when we come together in difficult times, a sense of excitement, commitment, and unification is created that results in "collective effervescence." While the concept is simple, it is often forgotten. As Carrington says, "Imagine what

it would look like in our schools (and communities) if we created more collective effervescence?" (p. 190).

- *"Lean In"* (p. 192). Bring the best version of yourself to work every day. Show up every day as authentically as possible and give the best of yourself to share your strengths and successes. Don't forget the impact you have made, and lean in to share with others around the table the way you got there. Do not shortchange yourself, as you have something important to say (p. 192).

Closing Thoughts

When it comes right down to it, we all know that nobody needs anything more added to their plates. Leaders, you are where you are because you too are amazing, and you excel at what you do. But when it comes to mental wellness, we leaders need to stop, or rather, pause. Because we all know that a principal's job is 24/7 and, dare I say it, 365 days a year. We need to breathe. We need to do check-ins on one another. It's just not easy to do. I can tell you from my own lived experience that it's worth it. Make your well-being and that of your staff a priority. It will pay off exponentially.

Moving forward, the question I leave you with is this: Am I working toward a flourishing, well school that focuses on the minds, hearts, and spirits of everyone in my care, including me?

For me, the answer is clear. After a great deal of "in-searching" and researching, I learned that there cannot be any other focus if the heart, mind, and spirit are not well. (In-searching is a term I learned many years ago from an Indigenous leader, Renée McGurry. It describes that deep philosophical digging that we do in our own heads and hearts.) I will continue to lead with the conviction to make my school the healthiest and strongest it can be by making workplace wellness a priority. As for the rest ... well, I can almost guarantee it all will fall into place!

Reflect and Respond

Take a moment to reflect on the following questions:

How will you focus on the mental wellness of your staff and yourself? What are you willing to commit to without stressing yourself out more as a leader? Are you willing to try one of the activities suggested in this chapter? How will you move forward? What will you do for yourself and others in times when you must be the calm in the chaos?

After completing your reflection, respond to the following:

- I am willing to commit to _____.
- I would like to talk to other leaders about _____.
- Someone that I consider a mentor that can help me with exploring this further is _____.
- What can I, as a leader, add to my "tool kit" to promote workplace wellness?

References and Further Reading

Beard, C. (2022, May 24). How to reset the button on your life: The wellness wheel exercise. *The blissful mind*. https://theblissfulmind.com/hit-the-reset-button/

Carrington, J. (2020). *Kids these days: A game plan for (re)connecting with those we teach, lead, & love*. Impress Books.

Crippen, C. (2005, December 5). The democratic school: First to serve, then to lead. *The Canadian Journal of Educational Administration and Policy, 47*. https://eric.ed.gov/?id=EJ846732

———. (2010). Serve, teach, and lead: It's all about relationships. *InSight: A Journal of Scholarly Teaching, 5*, 27–36.

Crippen, C., & Willows, J. (2019). Connecting teacher leadership and servant leadership: A synergistic partnership. *Journal of Leadership Education, 18*(2), 171–80. https://journalofleadershiped.org/jole_articles/connecting-teacher-leadership-and-servant-leadership-a-synergistic-partnership/

Douglas, L. (2020, November 23). *How to handle stress as a school principal*. Thrive. https://thriveglobal.com/stories/how-to-handle-stress-as-a-school-principal/

Hu, J., He, W., & Zhou, K. (2020). The mind, the heart, and the leader in times of crisis: How and when COVID-19-triggered mortality salience relates to state anxiety, job engagement, and prosocial behavior. *Journal of Applied Psychology, 105*(11), 1218–33. https://doi.org/10.1037/apl0000620

Johnson, B., & Bowman, H. (2021). *Dear teacher: 100 days of inspirational quotes and anecdotes*. Routledge.

Katz, J. (2012). *Teaching to diversity: The three-block model of universal design*. Portage & Main Press.

King, V. (2018). *Good vibes, Good life*. Hay House.

Kitchener, B. A., & Jorm, A. F. (2002). Mental health first aid training for the public: evaluation of effects on knowledge, attitudes and helping behavior. *BMC psychiatry*, 2, 10. https://doi.org/10.1186/1471-244x-2-10

Kowalchuk, T. (2014, November 25). School mental health: Not just about students anymore. *The Principal in Practice*. https://thomaskowalchuk.edublogs.org/2014/11/25/school-mental-health-not-just-about-students-any-more/

LifeWorks. (2021). *Workplace Mental Health Leadership*™ *certificate program*. https://lifeworks-learning.com/program/workplace-mental-health-leadership-certificate-program/

Rivkin, W., Diestel, S., & Schmidt, K-H. (2014, February 1). The positive relationship between servant leadership and employees' psychological health: A multi-method approach. *German Journal of Human Resource Management: Zeitschrift für Personalforschung, 28*(1–2), 57–72. https://journals.sagepub.com/doi/abs/10.1177/239700221402800104?journalCode=gjha

Rocco, M. (2020, February 5). Servant leadership: An ideal approach to enhance job satisfaction in employees. *ETech: Playing by the Rules*. https://www.etechgs.com/blog/servant-leadership-enhance-job-satisfaction-in-employees/

Schroeder, B. (2016). The effectiveness of servant leadership in schools from a Christian perspective. *BU Journal of Graduate Studies in Education, 8* (2), 13–18.

Siegel, D. (n.d.). *Name it to tame it* [Video, 4:20]. YouTube. https://www.youtube.com/watch?v=ZcDLzppD4Jc

Seligman, M. (2018). PERMA and the building blocks of well-being. *The Journal of Positive Psychology, 13*(4), 333–35. https://doi.org/10.1080/17439760.2018.1437466

Spears, L. (2018). *Ten characteristics of a servant-leader*. Spears Center for Servant-Leadership. https://www.spearscenter.org/46-uncategorised/136-ten-characteristics-of-servant-leadership

Chapter 13

An Invitation for Leaders in Education

Creating Psychologically Safe Work Environments

Jennifer E. Lawson with Megan Hunter,
Shannon Gander, and Kelsey McDonald

My first principalship was at an inner-city elementary school in an economically disadvantaged community, where I was tasked with leading a staff of 30 and a student body of 350 children. Every day, this staff showed up and gave their hearts and souls to ensure that we provided these students with the best education possible. They created a safe and loving environment where students could thrive and find enjoyment in the pursuit of learning.

I was so very proud of this team, and I was always trying to find ways to express that pride daily. Initially, I did what was mentored to me. When I was a new teacher in the inner city, my principal had a wonderful routine of "doing the rounds" with the vice principal every morning and afternoon to visit each classroom. This had a positive impact on the school. The students loved the visits, teachers felt acknowledged and proud, and the administration presented as a united team. So, when I became a principal, I simply did what came naturally to me. That was to treat the staff the way I wanted to be treated when I was a teacher. We all thrive on positive feedback and support, so I visited every classroom every day so that I could celebrate the good work the staff was doing—and tell them so. I found other ways to acknowledge staff, including providing personal feedback. I carried a pad of sticky notes wherever I went so that I could write a quick note and pop it in a staff member's mailbox, just to say, "Thank you," or "Well done!" I continued this practice over the years because staff regularly told me that it was empowering, affirming, and rewarding.

Yet I didn't know if I was doing enough. I was always looking for what else I could do to serve and support my staff. I'm sure that anyone in a leadership role within a school can identify with this. At times, when I worried about this, I also wondered what my staff was worried about. When I wasn't sleeping well, were they doing the same, wondering what more they could do for their students? Did they feel well supported by me?

I was fortunate to have a very cohesive team. I can't take all the credit for this. As colleagues, they were committed to supporting each other. We understood the importance of being a caring community where we focused on trust and enjoying each other's company. The staff room was a place of belonging. The office was often echoing with laughter. Even staff meetings typically reflected a sense of positive energy. We were in tune with each other in the passionate purpose of our work.

Of course, this does not mean that we didn't experience conflict or challenges. When things get tough, it is hard to always be positive and proactive. When teachers are burned out, through no fault of their own, it is very difficult for them to have the energy to support each other. At such times, we have a particular responsibility as leaders to encourage self-care for our staff. We need to offer resources to assist them on their wellness journeys. And we must find ways to take care of ourselves—something that is not easy to do but is so important to model.

Worldwide, administrators and school leaders are trying to figure out how to prevent educator burnout, support teachers to be well, and create a school community of wellness. Navigating an unforeseen pandemic with uncertain outcomes and increased rates of stress and mental health concerns has heightened this need.

I would bet my life that you are already engaging in actions to support educator wellness and a healthy school community. Whether you are a formal or informal leader, you are probably in constant conversation with your colleagues about how to create an environment of well-being in your school. That conversation likely extends to your family and friends outside of school. Plus you no doubt have your own "conversations" with yourself.

Fortunately, we happen to have more information about workplace well-being than ever to help us better understand the factors that affect psychological health and safety in the workplace. We can borrow from this well-researched information and embed these factors into our school culture as a systems-level approach to well-being.

Psychological Health and Safety in the Workplace

Canada is one of the first nations to develop psychological health and safety standards for promoting and protecting workplace well-being. Occupational health and safety standards exist to protect physical health. Psychological health and safety standards were developed as workplace safety criteria for the promotion and protection of psychological—including mental—health. In Canada, the development of these standards came about through a partnership between the Mental Health Commission of Canada (MHCC) and Canadian Safety Standards. The new standard has been in place since 2013 (MHCC, 2018).

The National Standard of Canada for Psychological Health and Safety in the Workplace (the Standard) describes 13 psychosocial factors that are known to impact psychological health in the workplace. Addressing these factors effectively can build the foundations of psychological protection and promotion in the workplace (Guarding Minds at Work, 2020).

You may already have addressed, or at least begun to tackle, many of these psychosocial factors in your school, division, or district. We know that having staff who are psychologically protected creates a workplace where people care for one another and one that promotes overall health and well-being. This, in turn, is passed along to the students who then receive a quality education from adults whose psychological well-being is prioritized.

Each of the 13 psychosocial factors listed in the Standard connects in obvious ways to our educational workplaces. These factors are listed below, along with some examples of stories from this book where these factors have been effectively addressed.[1]

---

1   The information in this section relies on these sources: CMHA Kelowna, 2022; Guarding Minds at Work, 2020, and Mental Health Commission of Canada, 2018.

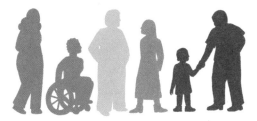

Psychological and Social Support

Civility and Respect

Clear Leadership and Expectations

Organizational Culture

Balance

INVOLVEMENT AND INFLUENCE

Psychological Protection

Workload Management

Protection of Physical Safety

Engagement

Psychological Competencies and Demands

Growth and Development

Recognition and Reward

Thirteen Psychosocial Factors

1. *Psychological and Social Support* is evident in a work environment where coworkers and supervisors are supportive of employees' psychological and mental health concerns and respond appropriately. The more employees feel they have psychological support, the greater their job attachment, job commitment, job satisfaction, job involvement, work mood, desire to remain with the organization, and job performance. As an example, in chapter 7, "Finding Joy(ce)," psychological support made all the difference for Joyce. In her story, she shares how supportive her principal was and how the school division's wellness resources were part of her recovery.

   In addition, offering professional development can help educators identify when a colleague is struggling and equip them with some resources to support them. Good options are Mental Health First Aid (offered by the MHCC, at: https://www.mhfa.ca/>) or training for all staff on the 13 psychosocial factors. Offering specific training to leaders and whole staff groups will ensure higher levels of competency system-wide.

2. *Organizational Culture* refers to the degree to which a work environment is characterized by trust, honesty, and fairness. "Fairness" means based on equity—we all get what we need even if it's not the same because we all have different needs as individuals. Organizational trust is essential to positive and productive social processes in any workplace. Trust is a predictor of cooperative behaviour, organizational citizenship behaviours, organizational commitment, and employee loyalty—all of which help retain and attract employees. In chapter 10, "Bringing Our Voices Together," Monika and North Star explore the importance of trust, both as colleagues and with their class of students. This trust was the foundation of their positive and safe relationships.

3. *Clear Leadership and Expectations* are apparent in a work environment where there are effective leaders who help employees know what they need to do and how their work contributes to the organization, and who inform and support them when there are impending changes. This increases employee morale, resiliency, and trust and decreases employee frustration and conflict. In chapter 12, "The Principal's Principles," Sandra conveys how school leadership, and more specifically servant leadership, can intentionally promote and foster a culture of wellness. She emphasizes the importance of being a strong communicator and helping staff to understand their value in the team and school community.

4. *Civility and Respect* in the workplace mean that staff are considerate in their interactions with one another, as well as with students, families, and the public. A civil and respectful workplace is linked to greater job satisfaction, greater perceptions of fairness, a more positive attitude, and improved morale. It also signals better teamwork, greater interest in personal development, engagement in problem resolution, enhanced supervisor-staff relationships, and a reduction in sick leave and turnover. Chapter 8, "Building Relationships for Well-Being," presents some important insights on how our thoughts, choices, and actions affect our interpersonal dynamics and how we navigate conflict in our school community.

5. *Psychological Competencies and Demands* are evident in a work environment where there is a good fit between employees' interpersonal and emotional competencies and the requirements of the position they hold. This is sometimes

referred to as psychological job fit. It is associated with fewer physical health complaints, lower levels of depression, greater self-esteem, and a more positive self-concept.

Matching the right person with the right job is important. It's about being hired based not only on your knowledge and background fitting the job but also on having the emotional and psychological skills to do it. It also involves continually being supported through training, personal and professional development, and coaching so that staff are successful on the job. Support could mean, for example, ensuring that a principal gets leadership training rather than just moving from a classroom teacher role into an administrator role with the assumption that the skills and psychological preparedness will follow.

6. *Growth and Development* are apparent in a work environment where employees receive encouragement and support in the development of their interpersonal, emotional, and job skills. Employee development increases goal commitment, organizational commitment, and job satisfaction. Such workplaces provide a range of internal and external opportunities for employees to build their range of competencies. This will not only help their current jobs but also prepare them for possible future positions.

    In chapter 11, Kelsey shares some powerful stories of how educators grow and develop alongside their colleagues. For example, when Kelsey was a new teacher, her principal selected the school counsellor, Sherry, to be her mentor. Sherry had specific expertise in the areas of growth and development that Kelsey needed. Kelsey's pedagogy was strong, but her repertoire of classroom management skills was not extensive enough to meet the social-emotional learning needs of her students. Sherry helped Kelsey learn how to identify students' emotions and foster calm over chaos. Kelsey was subsequently able to support Claire, another new classroom teacher. These powerful growth opportunities served Kelsey well throughout her career as a classroom teacher, counsellor, and principal.

7. *Recognition and Reward* are seen in a work environment where there is appropriate acknowledgement and appreciation of employees' efforts in a fair and timely manner. Recognition and reward together can motivate employees, fuel their desire to excel, build their self-esteem, encourage them

to exceed expectations, and enhance team success. This includes appropriate and regular financial compensation, as well as employee or team celebrations, recognition of years served, and milestones reached. Frequent, small gestures of appreciation can help employees feel valued more than waiting until major milestone celebrations. The "Post-it note" practice is an example of a low-tech, subtle, and yet high-impact way to recognize and celebrate staff.

8. *Involvement and Influence* occur when employees are included in discussions about how their work is done and how important decisions are made. When employees feel they have meaningful input into their work, they are more likely to be engaged, have higher morale, and take pride in their organization. It's important that we avoid making decisions on behalf of our educators without involving them when they will ultimately be the ones to carry out the decision that was made. As a recent example, consider the toll on educators for over two years during the pandemic, when they had little control and involvement in decision-making. It follows that school leaders now, more than ever, consider genuine efforts to engage school staff as an important step in building trust, promoting pride, and reviving passion.

9. *Workload Management:* Employee mental health benefits from a work environment where tasks and responsibilities can be accomplished within the time available. Having too much to do in too little time is the psychosocial factor that many working Canadians describe as being the biggest workplace stressor. In chapter 2, our authors encourage us to give ourselves permission to be well. They aim to empower us to take care of ourselves with kindness and compassion. We must acknowledge and redefine the pressures of strenuous workloads. As leaders, we have to demonstrate that we have the backs of our teachers. This requires us to set boundaries where we can. It also means being strategic when starting new initiatives, rather than taking on every new program and project (when the cost is educator burnout and turnout that affects the whole school community).

10. *Engagement* is evident in a work environment where employees feel connected to their work and are motivated to do their job well. This results in higher productivity for the employee and higher success for the organization.

Employee engagement also enhances job performance as well as morale and motivation. As leaders, we can sometimes settle into a pattern of turning to the same employees to get our needs met. Perhaps these are staff who quickly say yes, take on extra work, and don't ask many questions. The impact of this is disharmony in a team. Staff who feel left out and disconnected from you, as their leader, and the rest of the team, are disengaged. Lack of engagement leads to burnout, which we are always trying to mitigate. Use your awareness as a leader to take inventory of how you are spreading the work and the opportunities. Ensure that you are engaging employees throughout your entire school community.

11. *Balance* is seen in a work environment where the need for balance between the demands of work, family, and personal life is recognized. A healthy work-life balance makes employees feel valued and happier both at work and at home. Balance reduces stress and the possibility that home issues will spill over into work, or vice versa. Having work-life harmony and balance allows for time to attend to, for example, physical well-being, as outlined in chapter 5. In many of the stories in this book, writers share the impact of a lack of balance they experienced at some point in their teaching careers.

12. *Psychological Protection* occurs in a work environment where employees' psychological safety is ensured. This is evident when workers feel able to put themselves on the line, ask questions, seek feedback, report mistakes and problems, or propose a new idea without fearing negative consequences. When employees are psychologically protected, they demonstrate greater job satisfaction, have enhanced team learning behaviour, and improved performance. In chapter 1, we explored servant leadership, an approach in which a leader serves their staff in a way that helps them thrive. The characteristics of a servant-leader include empathy and listening, both of which enhance a leader's ability to create psychological protection for staff.

13. *Protection of Physical Safety* is established in a work environment where management takes appropriate action to protect the physical safety of employees. Employees who perceive the workplace as protecting physical safety will feel more secure and engaged at work. Research has shown that when employees

have higher levels of confidence in safety protection at work, they experience lower rates of psychological distress and mental health problems. There is no doubt that empowering staff to flourish begins with the establishment of physical safety for all. This becomes the foundation for all other forms of support.

Interestingly, I had never heard of these standards for psychological health and safety in the workplace while working as a principal, university instructor, or school trustee. I certainly recognize that, in all three arenas, many of the standards were being met due to efforts to maintain a positive school culture. However, now I also understand the importance of learning about and intentionally fostering these standards in our schools and school systems.

Again, I have no doubt that administrators everywhere are engaging in actions to effectively address these workplace factors for educators in their school communities. We can continue to seek out the good information and resources available to us on actions that further foster better workplaces and guidance on how leaders can incorporate psychological health and safety practices into their professional practice.

Here are some valuable resources about psychological health and safety standards and their implementation in the workplace:

- Guarding Minds at Work: <https://www.guardingmindsatwork.ca/>.
- Workplace Strategies for Mental Health: <https://www. workplacestrategiesformentalhealth.com/>.
- Canadian Mental Health Association Kelowna (CMHA Kelowna): <https://cmhakelowna.com/13-factors/>. This website also includes educational videos on the Psychological Health and Safety Standards.
- Mental Health Commission of Canada, Mental Health First Aid Canada: <https://www.mhfa.ca/>.

Reflect and Respond

Take some time now to consider how the Standard for Psychological Health and Safety in the Workplace might be promoted in your school, division, or district.

- In what areas do you see psychological health and safety being fostered successfully in your school, division, or district?
- What actions might you take to further implement the Standard for Psychological Health and Safety in the Workplace?
- You may want to share this information on workplace factors affecting psychological health and safety with others in your workplace. Who would you choose? Colleagues, senior administration, acquaintances who are leaders in other organizations?
- How might you further promote the Standard?

References and Further Reading

Canadian Mental Health Association Kelowna. (2022). *13 psychosocial factors for psychological health and safety in the workplace.* https://cmhakelowna.com/13-factors/

Guarding Minds at Work. (2020). *Know the psychosocial factors.* https://www.guardingmindsatwork.ca/about/about-psychosocial-factors

Mental Health Commission of Canada. (2018). *National Standard.* https://mentalhealthcommission.ca/national-standard/

Conclusion

Jennifer E. Lawson

It is our sincere hope that this book has provided you with an opportunity to reflect on your own well-being as much as the well-being of your colleagues and students. The stories, journeys, and strategies presented here may help us to reflect on our common humanity and foster positive mental health for ourselves and those in our lives. We all have times of great joy, great sadness, and great stress. Our wish for you is that you find the balance that allows you to live your life in a way that is comfortable, healthy, and happy.

We encourage you to reflect on the Sacred Hoop to examine your current experience of balance and well-being. Do this without judgment (no matter where you are at) or comparison to what others are doing. Be curious when considering what you need at this time. Curiosity fosters hope and helps us to remain open to new possibilities.

We are grateful to Elder Kipling and Knowledge Keeper North Star for sharing their perspectives throughout this book. To end our wellness journey together, we look to their thoughts on how the Sacred Hoop can help us move forward.

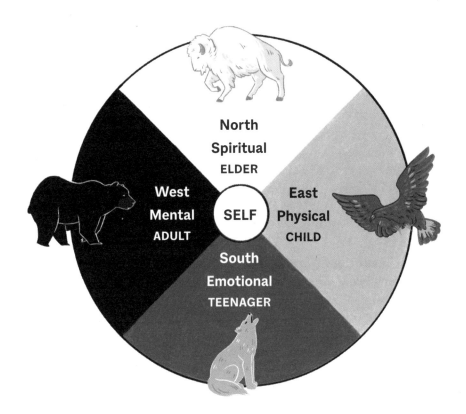

North
Spiritual
ELDER

West
Mental
ADULT

SELF

East
Physical
CHILD

South
Emotional
TEENAGER

One of the many teachings of the Sacred Hoop is about achieving balance or well-being in life. We must constantly strive to find this harmony, while also knowing that balance can only be achieved for short periods of time, and then something goes out of balance. So we must constantly be self-aware, carefully observing and feeling what is happening within us and around us, so we can be prepared to address our wellness needs.

Once around the Sacred Hoop is not enough, nor is one teaching from the Sacred Hoop. On our journeys to positive mental health and well-being, we will sometimes need to go back to the teachings we have already explored to rehear, relearn, and refocus.—*Elder Kipling*

We have heard the voices of each educator who has shared their wellness journey. The path forward is not often a straight path, but one with curves, bumps, and obstacles. The Sacred Hoop offers us a route toward wellness that is not always clear or free from challenges. Our wellness journey, like the Sacred Hoop, is never truly over. It is more a circle that we will continually walk. There is no destination. We journey around the Sacred Hoop again and again, while with each step, we add new understanding about wellness and let go of things that no longer serve us.

There will be times when we feel lonely and isolated in our profession. Remember that we all belong inside the Circle. We cannot face this journey alone. Together we are better for being of service to others, as we grow in understanding our personal and collective wellness journeys. Mino Pimatisiwin means "living a good life." It means walking in a good way and learning from how others walk their walk. It has been my pleasure to walk beside you. I've enjoyed journeying around the Sacred Hoop, learning more about others and myself in deeper and more meaningful ways. Miigwech for allowing me on your sacred walk.—*North Star*